ENDOMORPH DIET COOKBOOK FOR BEGINNERS

Easy delicious recipes including meal plan, health benefits, nutritional value and more!

Esther Harts

TABLE OF CONTENTS

The endomorph body type is one of the three primary body types, alongside the ectomorph and mesomorph. Endomorphs typically have a rounder, softer appearance, with a higher body fat percentage. They tend to have a slower metabolism and may find it easier to gain weight, especially in the form of fat.

Characteristics of an Endomorph

1. **Round Body Shape:** Endomorphs usually have a rounder body shape, with wider hips and shoulders. They often have shorter limbs and a softer, rounder appearance overall.

2. **Higher Body Fat Percentage:** Endomorphs tend to have a higher percentage of body fat compared to ectomorphs and mesomorphs. This can make it more challenging for them to lose weight and maintain a lean physique.

3. **Slower Metabolism:** Endomorphs typically have a slower metabolism, which means they burn

calories at a slower rate than ectomorphs and mesomorphs. This can make it more difficult for them to lose weight, especially if they consume more calories than they burn.

Challenges of Being an Endomorph

1. **Weight Gain:** Endomorphs often find it easier to gain weight, especially in the form of fat. Even small changes in diet or exercise habits can lead to significant weight gain for endomorphs.

2. **Difficulty Losing Weight:** Because of their slower metabolism and higher body fat percentage, endomorphs may find it more challenging to lose weight than other body types. They may need to work harder and be more consistent with their diet and exercise routine to see results.

3. **Tendency to Store Fat:** Endomorphs tend to store fat more easily than other body types, especially around the abdomen, hips, and thighs. This can make it difficult to achieve a lean, toned physique.

4. **Struggle with Building Muscle:** While endomorphs may have an easier time building muscle compared to ectomorphs, they still may struggle to achieve a lean, toned appearance. They may need to focus on both strength training and cardiovascular exercise to achieve their fitness goals.

5. **Risk of Health Issues:** Carrying excess weight, especially around the abdomen, can increase the risk of health issues such as heart disease, diabetes, and high blood pressure. Endomorphs need to pay close attention to their diet and exercise habits to maintain a healthy weight and reduce their risk of these health problems.

CHAPTER 1

THE SCIENCE OF ENDOMORPH METABOLISM

Our bodies are all different, and one of the ways they differ is in how they process food and energy. This is often referred to as metabolism. Metabolism is the process through which your body transforms the food and beverages you consume into energy. The ectomorph, mesomorph, and endomorph are the three main body types. Each body type has its own unique metabolic characteristics.

1. **Ectomorphs:** Ectomorphs are typically thin with a fast metabolism. They have a hard time gaining weight and may find it difficult to put on muscle.

2. **Mesomorphs:** Mesomorphs have a more athletic build with a moderate metabolism. They tend to have an easier time gaining muscle and losing fat compared to ectomorphs and endomorphs.

3. **Endomorphs:** Endomorphs have a slower metabolism and tend to gain weight more easily. They may have a harder time losing fat and may need to be more careful about their diet and exercise habits.

Factors Influencing Endomorph Metabolism

1. **Genetics:** Genetics play a significant role in determining your metabolic rate and body type. Endomorphs may have inherited genes that predispose them to have a slower metabolism and store more fat.

2. **Hormones:** Hormones also play a crucial role in metabolism. Hormones like insulin, cortisol, and thyroid hormones can influence how your body processes food and energy. Endomorphs may have hormonal imbalances that affect their metabolism and make it harder for them to lose weight.

3. **Muscle Mass:** Muscle mass is another important factor in metabolism. Muscle tissue burns calories even when the body is at rest, unlike fat tissue. Therefore, individuals with higher muscle mass generally have a faster metabolism.

Endomorphs may have a harder time building and maintaining muscle mass, which can contribute to a slower metabolism.

4. **Diet and Exercise Habits:** Diet and exercise habits also play a significant role in metabolism. Endomorphs may need to pay closer attention to their diet and exercise routine to maintain a healthy weight and metabolism. They may need to focus on eating a balanced diet with plenty of fruits, vegetables, lean proteins, and whole grains, and incorporating regular exercise into their routine to boost their metabolism and burn more calories.

5. **Age:** Metabolism tends to slow down with age, which can make it harder to maintain a healthy weight, especially for endomorphs. As you get older, you may need to adjust your diet and exercise habits to accommodate these changes in metabolism.

CHAPTER 2

KEY PRINCIPLES OF ENDOMORPH DIET

For endomorphs, balancing macronutrients (carbohydrates, proteins, and fats) is crucial for managing weight and optimizing metabolism. Here's a breakdown of how endomorphs can balance their macronutrients effectively:

1. Carbohydrates
 - Focus on complex carbohydrates: Choose whole grains like brown rice, quinoa, oats, and whole wheat bread over refined grains like white rice and white bread.
 - Limit simple carbohydrates: Minimize sugary foods and drinks like soda, candy, and baked goods, as they can cause spikes in blood sugar levels and promote fat storage.

2. Proteins
 - Include lean protein sources: Opt for lean meats like chicken, turkey, and fish, as well as plant-based sources like beans, lentils, tofu, and tempeh.

- Protein helps to build and maintain muscle mass, which can help boost metabolism and support weight loss.

3. Fats
- Opt for healthy fats: Add nutritious fat sources to your diet, such as avocados, nuts, seeds, olive oil, and fatty fish such as salmon.
- Limit saturated and trans fats: Minimize intake of foods high in saturated and trans fats, such as fried foods, fatty cuts of meat, and processed snacks.

Optimizing Meal Timing and Frequency

1. Regular Meals
- Aim for three balanced meals every day, with snacks as required to maintain energy levels.
- Skipping meals can lead to overeating later in the day, so try to eat at regular intervals.

2. Breakfast
- Begin your day with a well-rounded breakfast containing protein, carbohydrates, and nutritious fats.
- Eating breakfast can kickstart your metabolism and prevent overeating later in the day.

3. Post-Workout Nutrition
 - Refuel your body with a combination of protein
and carbohydrates after exercise to support muscle
recovery and replenish energy stores.
 - A protein shake, yogurt with fruit, or a turkey
sandwich on whole grain bread are good
post-workout options.

Portion Control Strategies

1. Use Smaller Plates
 - Divide your plate, allocating half for vegetables, a
quarter for lean protein, and a quarter for whole
grains or starchy vegetables.
 - Divide your plate into halves, with one half filled
with vegetables, and the other half divided between
lean protein and whole grains or starchy vegetables.

2. Listen to Your Body
 - Pay attention to hunger and fullness cues, and
stop eating when you feel satisfied, not stuffed.
 - Eat slowly and savor your food to give your body
time to register feelings of fullness.

3. Be Mindful of Snacking

 - Opt for nutrient-rich snacks such as fruits, vegetables, nuts, and yogurt.
 - Portion out snacks into small containers or bags to avoid overeating.

4. Limit Liquid Calories

 - Be mindful of liquid calories from sugary drinks, alcohol, and high-calorie coffee beverages.
- Choose water, unsweetened tea, or sparkling water with a hint of fruit juice instead.

CHAPTER 3

FOOD CHOICES FOR ENDOMORPHS

Endomorphs often struggle with managing their weight due to their slower metabolism and tendency to store fat more easily. However, by focusing on nutrient-dense foods and making healthy choices, endomorphs can support their metabolism and achieve their fitness goals. Here are some of the best foods for endomorphs to include in their diet:

1. **Lean Proteins**
 - Chicken breast.
 - Turkey breast.
 - Fish (salmon, tuna, and trout).
 - Lean cuts of beef and pork (loin, sirloin).
 - Eggs.
 - Plant-based proteins (tofu, tempeh, legumes, lentils).

2. **Complex Carbohydrates**
 - Whole grains (brown rice, quinoa, oats, barley, whole wheat)
 - Sweet potatoes

- Legumes (beans, lentils, chickpeas)
  - Vegetables (broccoli, spinach, kale, Brussels sprouts, cauliflower)
  - Fruits such as berries, apples, oranges, bananas, and pears.

3. Healthy Fats
 - Avocado
 - Nuts (almonds, walnuts, pistachios)
 - Seeds like chia seeds, flaxseeds, and pumpkin seeds.
 - Olive oil
 - Fatty fish (salmon, mackerel, sardines)

4. Low-Fat Dairy
 - Greek yogurt
 - Skim milk
 - Cottage cheese
 - Reduced-fat cheese

5. Fiber-Rich Foods
 - Whole grains
 - Vegetables
 - Fruits
 - Legumes

These foods are nutrient-dense, meaning they provide essential vitamins, minerals, and antioxidants that support overall health and well-being. They also provide a good balance of carbohydrates, protein, and healthy fats, which can help regulate blood sugar levels, increase satiety, and support weight management.

Foods to Limit or Avoid

While it's important for endomorphs to focus on nutrient-dense foods, there are also some foods they should limit or avoid to support their health and fitness goals:

1. **Processed Foods**
 - Processed foods like chips, cookies, cakes, and other baked goods are often high in unhealthy fats, sugar, and calories but low in nutrients. They can contribute to weight gain and health problems like heart disease and diabetes.

2. **Sugary Foods and Beverages**
 - Foods and drinks high in added sugars, such as soda, candy, desserts, and sweetened beverages, can cause blood sugar spikes and promote fat storage.

3. High-Fat Foods

   - While healthy fats are an important part of a balanced diet, endomorphs should limit their intake of high-fat foods like fried foods, fatty cuts of meat, and full-fat dairy products, as they can contribute to weight gain and health problems.

4. Simple Carbohydrates

   - Foods made with refined grains, such as white bread, white rice, and pasta, should be limited, as they can cause blood sugar spikes and promote fat storage.

5. Alcohol

   - While moderate alcohol consumption is generally considered safe, excessive alcohol intake can contribute to weight gain and health problems, especially for endomorphs who are already prone to storing fat more easily.

CHAPTER 4

ENDOMORPH DIET PLAN

Here's a 21-day diet plan tailored for an endomorph body type. This comprises a variety of nutrient-rich foods to help in weight loss and promote health in general.

Day 1

Breakfast: Oatmeal with Nut Butter and Fruit.

Lunch: Turkey and Avocado Wrap.

Dinner: Grilled Steak, Baked Sweet Potato, and Asparagus.

Day 2

Breakfast: Greek Yogurt Parfait.

Lunch: Black Bean and Quinoa Salad.

Dinner: Shrimp and Vegetable Skewers with Quinoa.

Day 3

Breakfast: Egg and Vegetable Scramble.

Lunch: Tuna Salad Stuffed Avocado.

Dinner: Eggplant Parmesan with Whole Wheat Pasta.

Day 4

Breakfast: Smoothie with Protein Powder.

Lunch: Lentil Soup with Whole Grain Bread

Dinner: Mushroom and Spinach Stuffed Chicken Breast

Day 5

Breakfast: Veggie Omelette with Whole Grain Toast.

Lunch: Lentil and Sweet Potato Shepherd's Pie.

Dinner: Baked Cod, and Roasted-Brussels Sprouts with Cauliflower.

Day 6

Breakfast: Cottage Cheese and Fruit Plate.

Lunch: Quinoa together with Black Bean Stuffed Bell Peppers.

Dinner: Beef, and Broccoli Stir-Fry with Brown-Rice.

Day 7

Breakfast: Whole Grain Toast with Avocado.

Lunch: Greek Chicken Pita-Pocket with Tzatziki Sauce.

Dinner: Thai Basil Chicken with Brown Rice.

Day 8

Breakfast: Quinoa Breakfast Bowl

Lunch: Chicken and Vegetable Lettuce Wraps

Dinner: Teriyaki Tofu Stir-Fry with Brown Rice.

Day 9

Breakfast: Breakfast Burrito with Egg, Beans, and Avocado

Lunch: Zucchini Noodles together with Pesto and Grilled Shrimp

Dinner: Spaghetti Squash with Turkey Bolognese Sauce

Day 10

Breakfast: Chia Seed Pudding with Berries

Lunch: Turkey, and Vegetable Stir-Fry with Brown Rice.

Dinner: Ratatouille with Grilled Chicken.

Day 11

Breakfast: Whole Grain Waffles with Almond Butter, and Sliced Banana.

Lunch: Vegetable Stir-Fry with Tofu.

Dinner: Grilled Pork Tenderloin with Roasted Root Vegetables.

Day 12

Breakfast: Sweet Potato and Black Bean Breakfast Hash.

Lunch: Caprese Salad with Grilled Chicken.

Dinner: Lemon Garlic Shrimp with Spinach and Whole Grain Couscous.

Day 13

Breakfast: Protein Pancakes, Greek Yogurt and Berries.

Lunch: Grilled Chicken Salad.

Dinner: Vegetable and Chickpea Curry.

Day 14

Breakfast: Protein-packed Breakfast Bowl with Greek Yogurt, Nuts, and Berries.

Lunch: Vegetable & Lentil Curry with Brown Rice.

Dinner: Cauliflower Crust Pizza with Chicken and Vegetables.

Day 15

Breakfast: Whole Grain Bagel, Smoked Salmon & Cream Cheese.

Lunch: Grilled Shrimp and Vegetable Skewers with Brown Rice.

Dinner: Turkey and Vegetable Chili.

Day 16

Breakfast: Breakfast Quinoa with Almond Milk and Mixed Berries.

Lunch: Spinach with Feta Turkey Burger, and Sweet-Potato Fries.

Dinner: Grilled Chicken with Roasted Vegetables.

Day 17

Breakfast: Breakfast Bowl with Scrambled Tofu and Sautéed Vegetables.

Lunch: Salmon Quinoa Bowl.

Dinner: Chicken Caesar Salad with Whole Grain Croutons.

Day 18

Breakfast: Avocado and Egg Toast with Tomato Slices.

Lunch: Chickpea and Vegetable Buddha Bowl.

Dinner: Stuffed Bell Peppers.

Day 19

Breakfast: Almond Butter and Banana Smoothie Bowl.

Lunch: Lentil and Vegetable Stew.

Dinner: Quinoa-Stuffed Acorn Squash.

Day 20

Breakfast: Spinach and Feta Egg Muffins.

Lunch: Grilled Veggie Quesadillas with Guacamole.

Dinner: Turkey Meatballs with Zucchini Noodles.

Day 21

Breakfast: Veggie Breakfast Wrap with Scrambled Eggs and Avocado.

Lunch: Asian-Style Chicken and Vegetable Rice Bowl.

Dinner: Baked Salmon with Quinoa and Steamed Broccoli.

BREAKFAST RECIPES

Balancing macronutrients and eating nutrient-dense foods is essential for endomorphs to support their metabolism and manage their weight. Here are some meal plans for breakfast, that are designed with endomorphs in mind:

Oatmeal with Nut Butter and Fruit

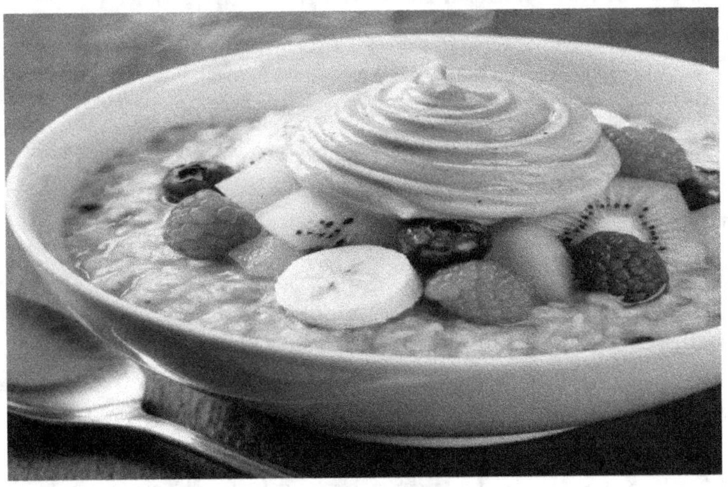

Ingredients:

1/2 cup rolled oats

1 cup water or milk (almond milk, soy milk, or regular milk)

1 tablespoon nut butter (almond butter, peanut butter, or cashew butter)

1/2 cup sliced fruits (banana, strawberries, blueberries, etc.)

1 teaspoon honey or maple syrup (optional)

Preparation Method:

In a small sauce-pan, boil the water or milk.

Stir in the rolled oats and reduce heat to medium-low.

Cook the oats, stirring occasionally, for about 5 minutes or until they reach your desired consistency.

Transfer the oats to a bowl once cooked.

Top the oatmeal with nut butter and sliced fruits.

Sprinkle it with honey or maple syrup if you want.

Cooking Time: Approximately 5 minutes

Nutritional Information:

Calories: 300-350 kcal

Protein: 8-10 grams

Fat: 10-15 grams

Carbohydrates: 45-50 grams

Fiber: 6-8 grams

Sugar: 10-15 grams.

Greek Yogurt Parfait

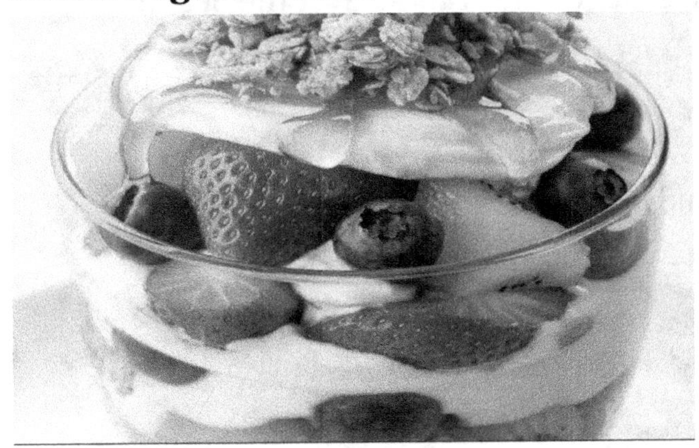

Ingredients:

- 1 container of Greek yogurt.

- 1/2 container blended berries (strawberries, blueberries, raspberries)

- 1/4 glass granola.

- 1 tablespoon nectar (optional).

Preparation:

1. Spoon half of the Greek yogurt into a glass.

2. Include half of the blended berries on best of the yogurt.

3. Drizzle half of the granola over the berries.

4. Rehash the layers with the remaining yogurt, berries, and granola.

5. Sprinkle with nectar, if desired.

Nutritional Information:

- Calories:Approximately 300 calories.

- Protein: **20g.**

- Fat: 7g.

- Carbohydrates: 40g.

- Fiber: 6g.

- Sugar: 24g.

- Sodium: 80mg.

Egg and Vegetable Scramble

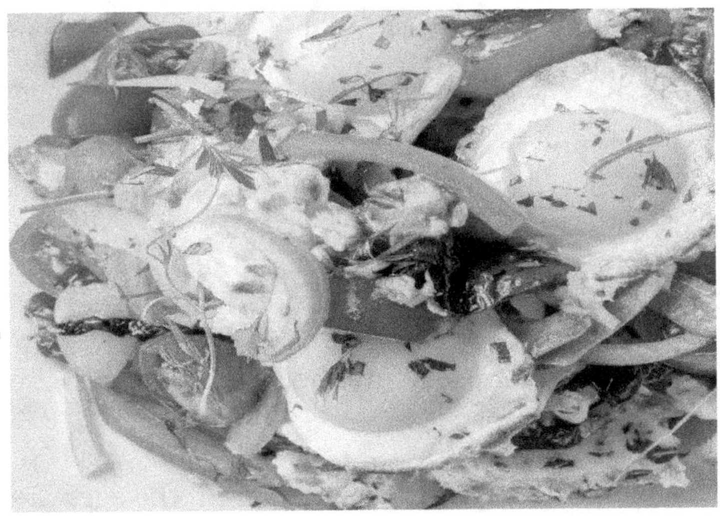

Ingredients:

- 2 eggs.

- 1/2 cup chopped vegetables (bell peppers, onions, spinach, mushrooms, etc.).

- 1 tablespoon of olive oil / cooking spray.

- Salt and pepper to taste.

- Optional: grated cheese, fresh herbs (like parsley or chives).

Preparation Method:

1. Put cooking spray or olive oil in a non-stick skillet over medium heat.

2. Add chopped vegetables to the skillet and sauté until they begin to soften, about 3-4 minutes.

3. In a bowl, beat the eggs with a pinch of salt and pepper.

4. Pour the beaten eggs into the frying-pan with the sautéed vegetables.

5. Stir continuously with a spatula until the eggs are fully cooked and scrambled, about 2-3 minutes.

6. If using, sprinkle grated cheese over the top of the scramble and allow it to melt for about 1 minute.

7. Take off the heat and add fresh herbs for garnish, if desired.

Cooking Time: Approximately 5-7 minutes.

Nutritional Information: (per serving)

- Calories: **220 kcal**

- Protein: **12g**

- Carbohydrates: **5g**

- Fat: **16g**

- Fiber: **2g**

- Sugar: **2g**

- Sodium: **320mg.**

Smoothie with Protein Powder

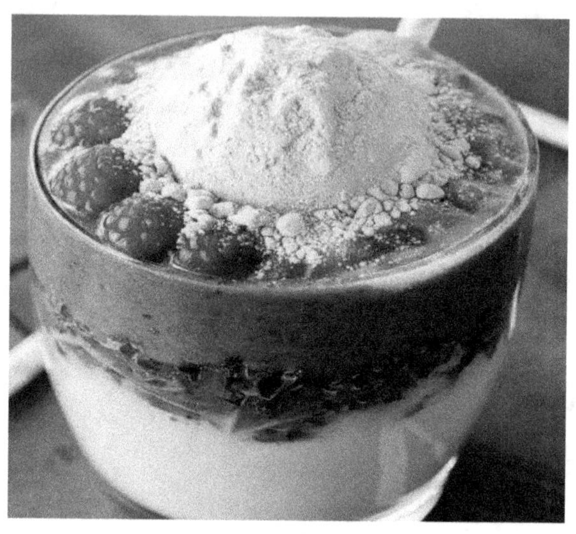

Ingredients:

- 1 cup spinach leaves

- 1 ripe banana

- 1 scoop protein powder (whey, pea, or hemp protein)

- 1 tablespoon chia seeds

-1 cup of your preferred milk, such as unsweetened almond milk.

- ½ cup plain Greek yogurt.

- Ice cubes (optional).

Preparation Method:

1. Add spinach leaves, banana, protein powder, chia seeds, Greek yogurt, and almond milk to a blender.

2. Blend at high speed until the mixture is smooth and creamy.

3. If desired, add ice cubes and blend again until smooth.

4. Pour into a glass cup and serve immediately.

Cooking Time:

- Preparation Time: 5 minutes.

- Total Time: 5 minutes.

Nutritional Information:

- Calories: Approximately 300 kcal.

- Protein: Approximately 25g.

- Carbohydrates: Approximately 35g.

- Fat: Approximately 8g.

- Fiber: Approximately 9g.

Veggie Omelette with Whole Grain Toast

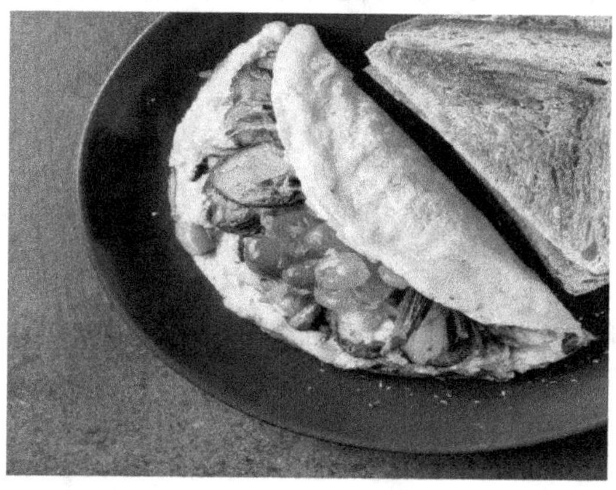

Ingredients:

For the omelet:

- 2 large eggs

- 1/4 cup of bell peppers, diced (any color).

- 1/4 cup diced onions.

- 1/4 cup chopped spinach

- Salt and pepper to taste

- 1 teaspoon of olive oil/ cooking spray.

- 2 slices whole grain bread.

- Butter or olive oil (optional).

Preparation:

1. In a bowl, whisk the eggs until well mixed. Season with salt and pepper.

2. Heat olive oil or cooking spray in a non-stick skillet over medium heat.

3. Add diced bell peppers and onions to the skillet. Cook for two to three minutes until they begin to soften.

4. Add chopped spinach to the skillet and cook for another 1-2 minutes until wilted.

5. Pour the beaten eggs over the vegetables in the skillet. Mix the skillet to distribute the eggs evenly.

6. Allow the omelette to cook undisturbed for 2-3 minutes, or until the edges start to set.

7. Carefully lift the edges of the omelet with a spatula and tilt the skillet to let any uncooked eggs flow to the edges.

8. Once the omelet is mostly set but still slightly runny on top, fold it in half using a spatula.

9. Cook for another 1-2 minutes until the omelet is cooked through but still moist inside.

For the whole grain toast:

1. Toast the whole grain bread until golden brown.

2. Spread with butter or drizzle with olive oil if desired.

Cooking Time:

- The omelet takes approximately 5-7 minutes to cook.

- The whole grain toast takes approximately 3-5 minutes to toast.

Nutritional Information:

- Calories: Approximately 300-350 calories (depending on the size of the eggs and amount of oil used).

- Protein: Approximately 15-20 grams

- Carbohydrates: Approximately 25-30 grams.

- Fat: Approximately 15-20 grams.

- Fiber: Approximately 5-7 grams.

Cottage Cheese and Fruit Plate

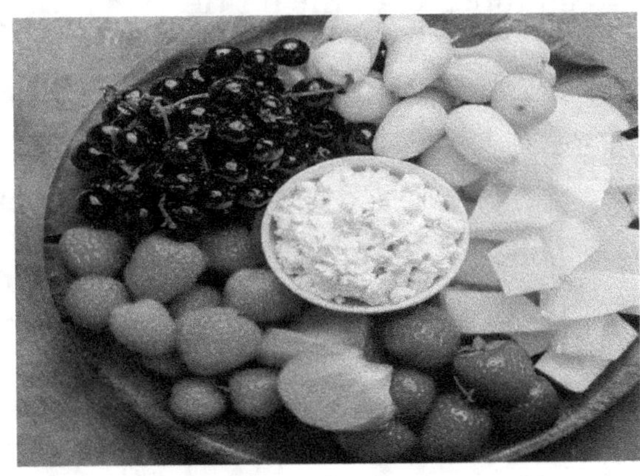

Ingredients:

- 1 cup low-fat cottage cheese.

- 1/2 cup of mixed berries (such as blueberries, strawberries or raspberries).

- 1/4 cup sliced almonds (optional).

- 1 teaspoon honey (optional).

Preparation Method:

1. Scoop the cottage cheese into a serving plate or bowl.

2. Arrange the mixed berries on top of the cottage cheese.

3. Sprinkle sliced almonds over the berries.

4. Drizzle honey over the top, if desired.

Nutritional Information:

- Servings: 1

- Calories: **Approximately 300 calories**

- Protein: **25g**

- Carbohydrates: **20g**

- Fat: **12g**

- Fiber: 5g

- Sugars: 14g.

Whole Grain Toast with Avocado

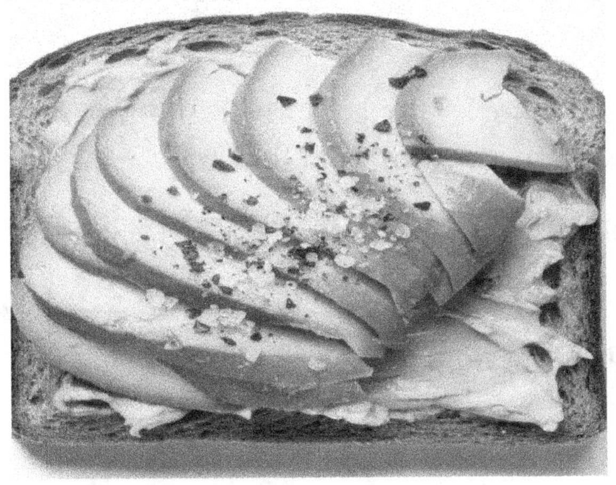

Ingredients:

- 2 slices of whole grain bread

- 1 ripe avocado

- 1 small tomato, sliced (optional)

- Salt and pepper to taste.

Preparation Method:

1. Toast the slices of whole grain bread until they are golden brown and crispy.

2. While the bread is toasting, cut the avocado in half, remove the pit, and scoop the flesh into a small bowl. Mash the avocado with a fork until it's smooth.

3. Once the toast is done, spread the mashed avocado evenly onto each slice of toast.

4. Top the avocado toast with sliced tomatoes if desired.

5. Season with salt and pepper to your taste.

Cooking Time:

- Toasting time: 3-5 minutes.

Nutritional Information:

- Calories: Approximately 250 calories per serving (2 slices of toast with 1 whole avocado)

- Total Fat: 15g

- Saturated Fat: 2g

- Trans Fat: 0 g

- Cholesterol: 0 mg

- Sodium: 150 mg

- Total Carbohydrates: 25 g

 - Dietary Fiber: 10 g

 - Sugars: 2g

- Protein: 5g.

Quinoa Breakfast Bowl

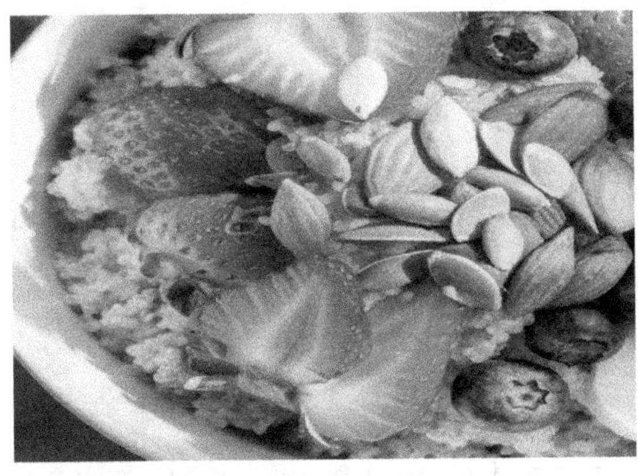

Ingredients:

- 1/2 cup quinoa.

- 1 cup almond milk.

- 1/2 teaspoon vanilla extract.

- 1/2 teaspoon ground cinnamon.

- 1 tablespoon maple syrup (optional).

- 1/2 cup mixed berries (e.g strawberries, blueberries, raspberries).

- 2 tablespoons chopped nuts (such as walnuts, almonds, or pecans).

- 1 tablespoon chia seeds (optional).

- Fresh mint leaves for garnish (optional).

Preparation:

1. Rinse the quinoa with cold water using a fine-mesh sieve.

2. In a small saucepan, combine the rinsed quinoa, almond milk, vanilla extract, and ground cinnamon.

3. Bring the mixture to a boil over medium heat, then reduce the heat to low and simmer, covered,

for 15-20 minutes, or until the quinoa is cooked and most of the liquid is absorbed.

4. Once cooked, fluff the quinoa with a fork and stir in the maple syrup, if using.

5. Divide the cooked quinoa into serving bowls.

6. Top each bowl with mixed berries, chopped nuts, and chia seeds.

7. Garnish with fresh mint leaves, if you want.

Cooking Time: 15-20 minutes.

Nutritional Information:

- Calories: Approximately 350-400 calories per serving (depending on added sweeteners and toppings).

- Protein: Approximately 10-12 grams.

- Carbohydrates: Approximately 50-55 grams.

- Fat: Approximately 12-15 grams.

- Fiber: Approximately 8-10 grams.

Breakfast Burrito with Egg, Beans, and Avocado

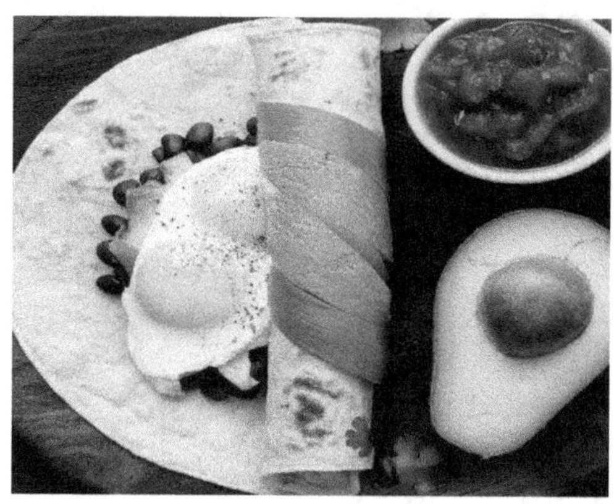

Ingredients:

- 2 large eggs

- 1/4 cup of black beans, washed and drained

- 1/4 avocado, sliced

- 1 whole wheat or spinach tortilla.

- Salt and pepper, to taste.

- Salsa (optional).

- Chopped cilantro (optional).

Preparation:

1. In a small bowl, beat the eggs with a pinch of pepper and salt.

2. Heat a non-stick skillet over medium heat and add the beaten eggs. Cook, stirring occasionally, until the eggs are cooked and scrambled throughout.

3. Warm the black beans in the microwave or on the stovetop.

4. Warm the tortilla in the microwave or on a skillet for about 10-15 seconds on each side.

5. Place the scrambled eggs, black beans, and avocado slices in the center of the tortilla.

6. Optional: Add salsa and chopped cilantro on top.

7. Fold the sides of the tortilla over the filling and roll it up tightly into a burrito.

Cooking Time:

- 10 minutes.

Nutritional Information:

- Calories: 380 kcal.

- Protein: 20g.

- Carbohydrates: 33g.

- Fat: 18g.

- Fiber: 10g.

- Sugar: 1g.

Chia Seed Pudding with Berries

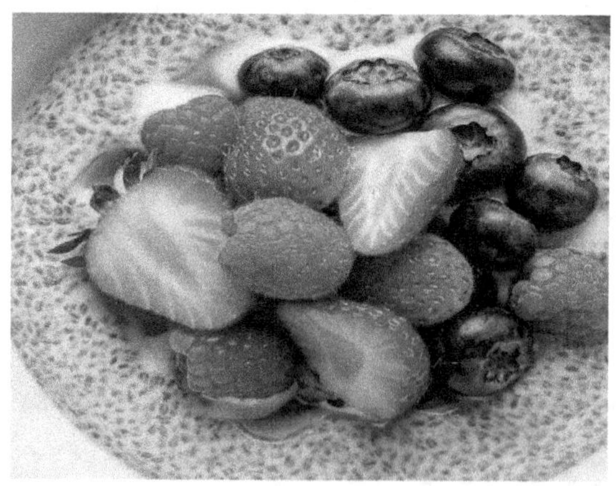

Ingredients:

- 1/4 cup chia seeds
- 1 cup of unsweetened almond milk or any milk of your choice.
- 1 tablespoon maple syrup or honey (if you want)
- 1/2 teaspoon vanilla extract
- 1/2 cup of mixed berries (strawberries, blueberries, raspberries).

Preparation Method:

1. In a bowl, mix together chia seeds, almond milk, maple syrup (if using), and vanilla extract. Stir well to combine.

2. Cover the bowl and refrigerate for at least 2 hours or over the night, so as to allow the chia seeds to absorb the liquid and form a pudding-like consistency. Stir occasionally during the first 30 minutes to prevent clumping.

3. Once the chia pudding has thickened, give it a final stir.

4. Serve the chia seed pudding in individual bowls or glasses, and top with mixed berries.

Cooking Time:

Preparation Time: 5 minutes

Chilling Time: 2 hours to overnight

Nutritional Information (per serving):

- Calories: 180 kcal.
- Protein: 6g.
- Fat: 9g.
- Carbohydrates: 20g.
- Fiber: 12g.
- Sugar: 6g.
- Calcium: 340mg.
- Iron: 3.5mg.
- Potassium: 250mg.

Whole Grain Waffles with Almond Butter and Sliced Banana

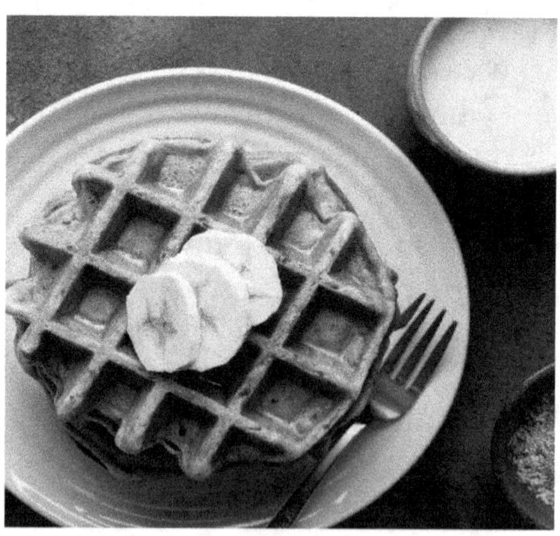

Ingredients:

- 1 cup whole wheat flour.

- 1 tablespoon baking powder.

- 1 tablespoon coconut sugar (optional).

- 1/4 teaspoon salt.

- 1 cup almond milk.

- 2 tablespoons of melted coconut oil / melted butter.

- 1 teaspoon vanilla extract.

- Almond butter.

- 1 banana, sliced.

Preparation:

1. Preheat your waffle iron according to the producer's instructions.

2. In a large mixing bowl, whisk together the whole wheat flour, baking powder, coconut sugar (if using), and salt.

3. In another bowl, whisk together the almond milk, melted coconut oil (or melted butter), and vanilla extract.

4. Pour the wet ingredients into the dry ingredients and stir until it is well mixed. Be careful not to overmix.

5. Lightly grease the waffle iron with coconut oil or non-stick cooking spray.

6. Pour enough batter onto the waffle iron to cover the waffle grids.

7. Close the lid and cook according to the manufacturer's instructions, usually about 3-5 minutes, or until the waffles are golden brown and crisp.

8. Repeat with the remaining batter.

Cooking Time:

- Approximately 3-5 minutes per batch, depending on your waffle iron.

Nutritional Information:(Per Serving)

- Calories: 330 kcal.

- Protein: 9g.

- Carbohydrates: 44g.

- Fat: 14g.

- Fiber: 6g.

- Sugar: 9g.

- Sodium: 486 mg.

Sweet Potato and Black Bean Breakfast Hash

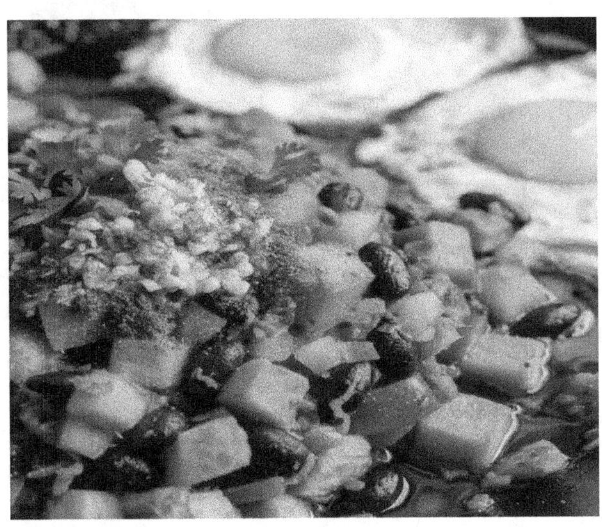

Ingredients:

- Two medium sweet potatoes, peeled and sliced into small pieces.

- 1 can (15 ounces) black beans, washed and drained

- 1 red bell pepper, diced

- 1 small onion, diced

- 2 cloves garlic, minced

- 1 teaspoon ground cumin

- 1 teaspoon smoked paprika

- Salt and pepper to taste

- 2 tablespoons olive oil

- 4 eggs (optional)

- Fresh cilantro, chopped (for garnish).

Preparation:

1. Heat the olive oil in a big frying pan over medium heat.

2. Add diced sweet potatoes to the skillet and cook, stirring occasionally, for about 5 minutes.

3. Add diced bell pepper and onion to the skillet and cook for another 5 minutes, or until vegetables are tender.

4. Add minced garlic, ground cumin, smoked paprika, salt, and pepper to the skillet. Stir well to combine.

5. Add black beans to the skillet and cook for an additional 2-3 minutes, until heated through.

6. If adding eggs, create small wells in the hash and crack an egg into each well. Cover the skillet and cook until the eggs are done to your preference.

7. Top with chopped fresh cilantro before serving.

Cooking Time: Approximately 20 minutes.

Nutritional Information:

(Per Serving, without eggs)

- Calories: 275 kcal.

- Protein: 8g.

- Fat: 7g.

- Carbohydrates: 45g.

- Fiber: 10g.

- Sugar: 7g.

- Sodium: 408mg.

Protein Pancakes with Greek Yogurt and Berries

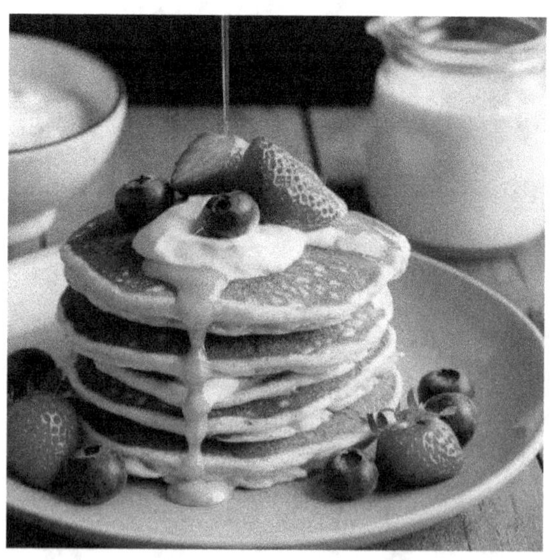

Ingredients:

- 1 scoop of protein powder (use the flavor of your choice).

- 1/2 cup rolled oats.

- 1/2 banana, mashed.

- 1/4 cup Greek yogurt.

- 1/4 cup almond milk (you can use any milk).

- 1 egg.

- 1/2 teaspoon baking powder.

- Cooking spray or oil for the pan.

For Serving:

- Greek yogurt.

- Fresh berries (such as strawberries, blueberries).

- Maple syrup or honey (optional).

Preparation:

1. In a blender, combine the rolled oats, banana, Greek yogurt, almond milk, egg, protein powder, and baking powder. Blend until smooth.

2. Heat a non-stick skillet or griddle over medium heat and coat it with cooking spray or a small amount of oil.

3. Pour 1/4 cup of the pancake batter onto the frying pan for each pancake. Cook until bubbles form on the surface of the pancake, flip and cook until it is golden brown on both sides.

4. Repeat with the remaining batter.

5. Serve the pancakes with a dollop of Greek yogurt, fresh berries, and a drizzle of maple syrup or honey if desired.

Cooking Time:

- Preparation Time: 5 minutes.

- Cooking Time: 10 minutes.

- Total Time: 15 minutes.

Nutritional Information: (per serving, without toppings)

- Calories: 350 kcal

- Protein: 30g

- Carbohydrates: 40g.

- Fat: 8g.

- Fiber: 6g.

- Sugar: 8g.

Protein-packed Breakfast Bowl with Greek Yogurt, Nuts, and Berries

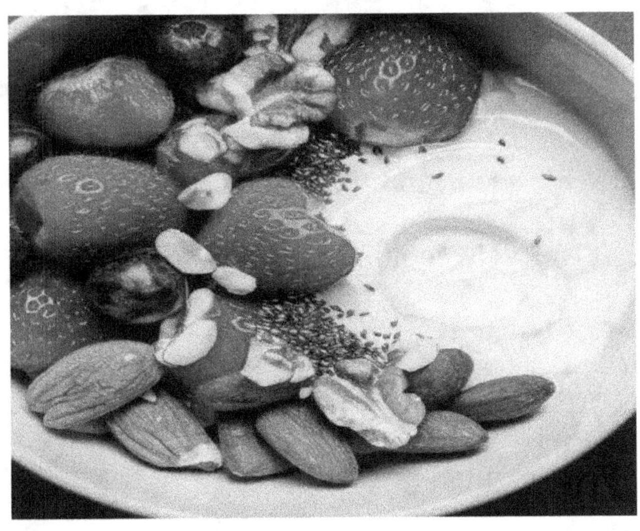

Ingredients:

- 1/2 cup Greek yogurt.

- 1/4 cup mixed nuts (almonds, walnuts).

- 1/4 cup mixed berries (strawberries, blueberries, raspberries).

- 1 tablespoon honey (optional).

- 1 tablespoon chia seeds (optional).

Preparation Method:

1. Place Greek yogurt in a bowl.

2. Top with mixed nuts and berries.

3. Drizzle honey over the top, if using.

4. Sprinkle chia seeds on top, if using.

Cooking Time: No cooking required.

Nutritional Information:

- Calories: **Approximately 300 kcal.**

- Protein: **Approximately 20g.**

- Carbohydrates: Approximately 20g.

- Fat: Approximately 15g.

- Fiber: Approximately 5g.

This breakfast bowl is high in protein, healthy fats, and fiber, making it a nutritious and filling option to start your day.

Whole Grain Bagel with Smoked Salmon and Cream Cheese

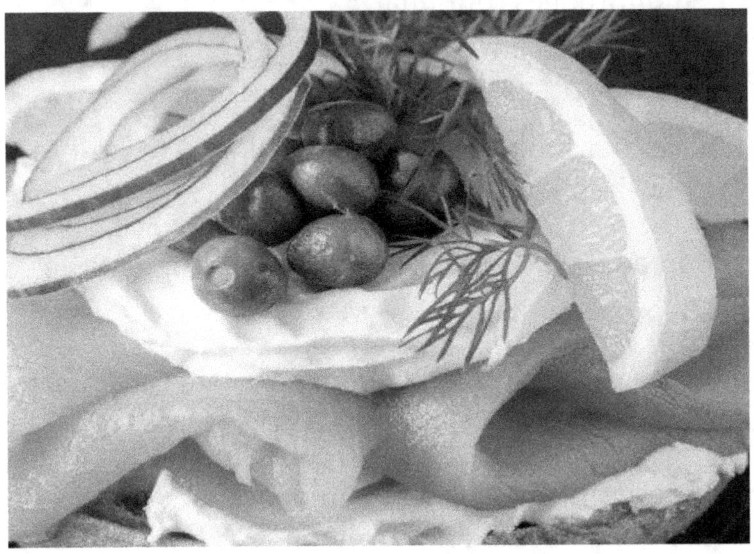

Ingredients:

- 1 whole grain bagel

- 50g smoked salmon

- 2 tablespoons cream cheese

- Sliced red onion (optional)

- Capers (optional)

- Fresh dill (optional)

- Lemon wedges (optional).

Preparation:

1. Slice the whole grain bagel in half and toast it to your desired level of crispness.

2. Spread cream cheese evenly on each half of the bagel.

3. Arrange the smoked salmon on top of the cream cheese.

4. If desired, add sliced red onion, capers, and fresh dill on top of the smoked salmon.

5. Serve with lemon wedges on the side.

Cooking Time:

- Preparation time: 5 minutes

- Cooking time: 5 minutes.

Nutritional Information:

- Calories: Approximately 350 kcal.

- Protein: Approximately 18g.

- Carbohydrates: Approximately 35g.

- Fat: Approximately 15g.

- Fiber: Approximately 6g.

Breakfast Quinoa with Almond Milk, and Mixed Berries

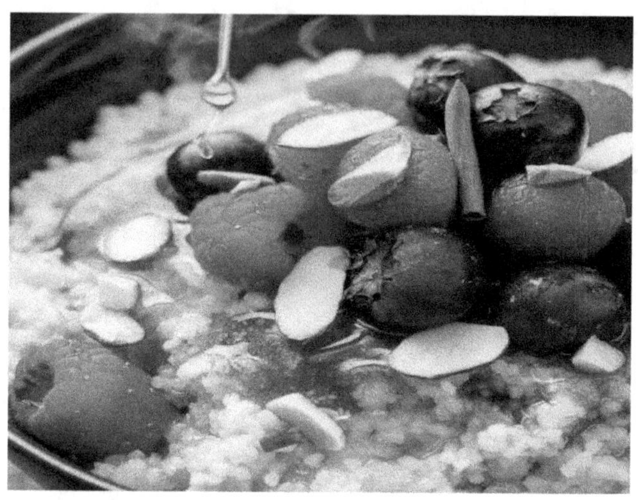

Ingredients:

- 1/2 cup quinoa

- 1 cup almond milk .

- 1 cup mixed berries (e.g strawberries, raspberries, blueberries).

- 1 tablespoon of honey.

- 1/4 teaspoon vanilla extract (optional)

- A pinch of cinnamon (optional)

- Sliced almonds or chopped nuts for garnish (optional).

Preparation Method:

1. Wash the quinoa under cold water in a fine-mesh sieve.

2. In a saucepan, combine the rinsed quinoa and almond milk.

3. Bring the mixture to a boil, then reduce the heat to low, cover, and simmer for about 15 minutes, or until the quinoa is tender and the liquid is absorbed. Stir occasionally.

4. Once the quinoa is cooked, remove it from the heat and let it sit, covered, for 5 minutes.

5. Fluff the quinoa with a fork and stir in the honey or maple syrup, vanilla extract, and cinnamon if using.

6. Divide the quinoa into serving bowls and top with mixed berries and sliced almonds or chopped nuts if desired.

Cooking Time: Approximately 20 minutes.

Nutritional Information

- Calories: Approximately 300 kcal per serving.

- Protein: Approximately 8g.

- Carbohydrates: Approximately 55g.

- Fat: Approximately 6g.

- Fiber: Approximately 7g.

- Sugar: Approximately 15g (depending on added sweeteners).

- Sodium: Approximately 170mg.

Breakfast Bowl with Scrambled Tofu and Sautéed Vegetables

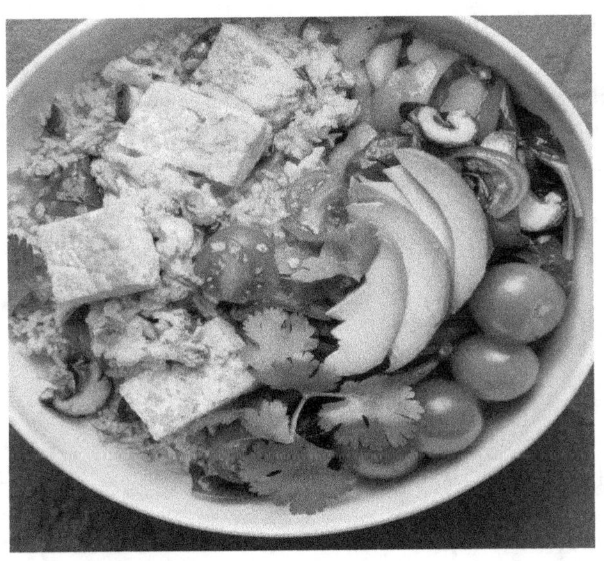

Ingredients:

For Scrambled Tofu:

- 200g firm tofu, crumbled.

- 1 tablespoon of olive oil.

- 1/4 teaspoon turmeric powder.

- Salt and pepper to taste.

For Sautéed Vegetables:

- 1/2 tablespoon olive oil.

- 1/2 cup sliced bell peppers.

- 1/2 cup sliced mushrooms.

- 1/4 cup diced onions.

- 1 cup fresh spinach leaves.

- Salt and pepper to taste.

For Breakfast Bowl:

- Cooked quinoa or brown rice

- Sliced avocado

- Cherry tomatoes, halved

- Fresh cilantro leaves for garnish.

Preparation:

1. Prepare Scrambled Tofu:

 - Heat the olive oil in a frying-pan over medium heat.

 - Add crumbled tofu to the skillet and sprinkle turmeric powder over it.

- Spice it with pepper and salt to taste.

- Cook, stirring occasionally, for 5-7 minutes or until tofu is heated through and slightly browned. Set aside.

2. Sauté Vegetables:

- Add olive oil, In the same skillet.

- Add sliced bell peppers, mushrooms, and onions to the skillet.

- Sauté for 5-7 minutes or until vegetables are tender.

- Add spinach leaves and cook for an additional 1-2 minutes until wilted.

- Dress it with pepper and salt to taste.

3. Assemble Breakfast Bowl:

- Divide cooked quinoa or brown rice into bowls.

- Top with scrambled tofu and sautéed vegetables.

- Add the sliced avocado and cherry tomatoes.

- Garnish with fresh cilantro leaves.

Cooking Time: Approximately 15 minutes.

Nutritional Information (per serving):

- Calories: 350 kcal.

- Protein: 15g.

- Carbohydrates: 30g.

- Fat: 20g.

- Fiber: 8g.

- Sugar: 4g.

- Sodium: 350mg.

Avocado and Egg Toast with Tomato Slices

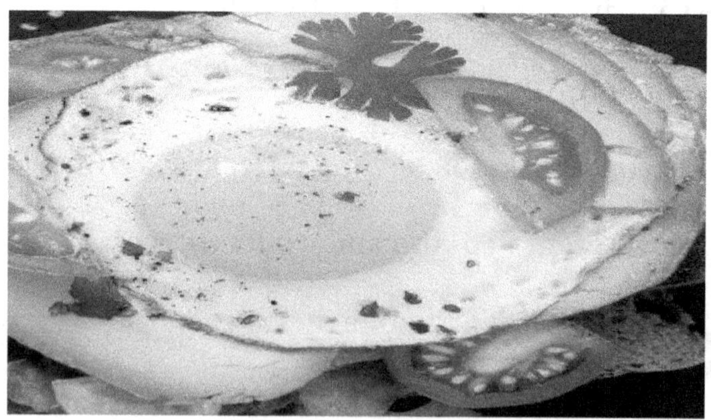

Ingredients:

- 1 ripe avocado

- 2 slices of whole grain bread

- 2 large eggs

- 1 medium tomato, thinly sliced

- Salt and pepper to taste

- Optional toppings: red pepper flakes, chopped cilantro, hot sauce.

Preparation:

1. Prepare the Avocado Spread:

 - Cut the avocado in half, remove the pit, and scoop the flesh into a small bowl.

 - Mash the avocado with a fork until smooth.

 - Season with pepper and salt to taste.

2. Cook the Eggs:

- Heat a non-stick frying pan over medium heat and spray with cooking spray or add a small amount of oil.

- Crack the eggs into the frying pan and cook to your desired doneness (fried, scrambled, or poached).

- Season with pepper and salt.

3. Toast the Bread:

- Toast the slices of the whole grain bread until golden brown.

4. Assemble the Toast:

- Spread the mashed avocado evenly on each of the toast.

- Add sliced tomato on top of each slice.

- Place the cooked eggs over the tomato slices.

- Spice with additional salt and pepper if desired.

- Garnish with optional toppings such as red pepper flakes, chopped cilantro, or hot sauce.

Cooking Time:

- Preparation: 5 minutes

- Cooking: 5 minutes.

Nutritional Information

(Per serving)

- Calories: **360 kcal.**

- Total Fat: **19g.**

  - Saturated Fat: **3.5g.**

  - Trans Fat: **0g.**

- Cholesterol: **370mg.**

- Sodium: **390mg.**

- Total Carbohydrate: **32g.**

  - Dietary Fiber: **9g.**

  - Sugars: **4g.**

- Protein: **18g.**

Almond Butter and Banana Smoothie Bowl

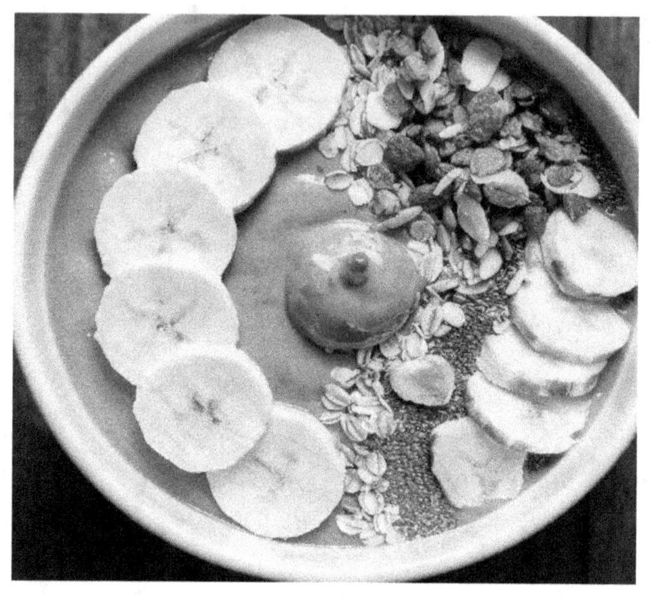

Ingredients:

- 1 ripe banana, sliced

- 2 tablespoons almond butter

- 1/2 cup unsweetened almond milk

- 1/4 cup rolled oats

- 1 tablespoon chia seeds

- 1/2 teaspoon vanilla extract

- Toppings: sliced banana, granola, sliced almonds, honey (optional).

Preparation:

1. In a blender, combine the sliced banana, almond butter, almond milk, rolled oats, chia seeds, and vanilla extract.

2. Blend until it's smooth and creamy. If needed, add more almond milk until it's the thickness you like.

3. Pour the smoothie into a bowl.

4. Top with sliced banana, granola, sliced almonds, and a drizzle of honey if desired.

Cooking Time:

- Preparation Time: 5 minutes.

Nutritional Information:

- Calories: 450.

- Protein: 11g.

- Carbohydrates: 56g.

- Fat: **22g.**

- Fiber: **10g.**

- Sugar: **22g.**

Spinach and Feta Egg Muffins

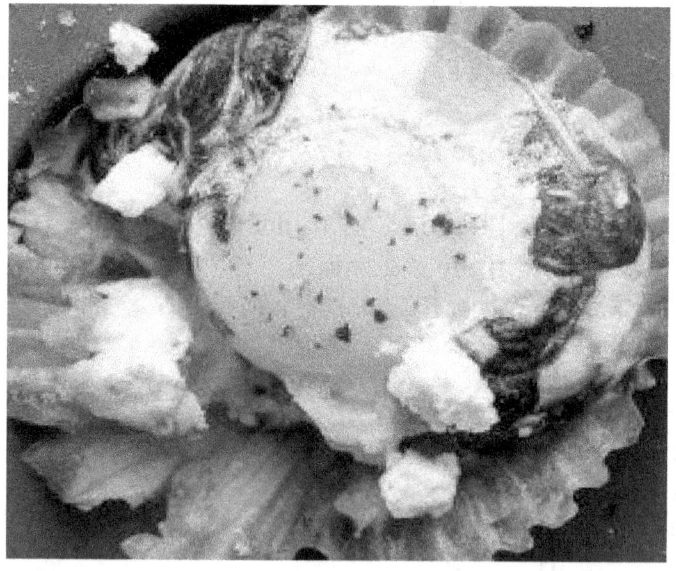

Ingredients:

- 8 large eggs.

- 1 cup chopped fresh spinach.

- 1/2 cup crumbled feta cheese.

- 1/4 cup diced red bell pepper.

- 1/4 cup diced onion.

- Salt and pepper to taste.

- Cooking spray or olive oil to grease the muffin tin.

Preparation Method:

1. Preheat your oven to 350°F (175°C). Coat a muffin tin with cooking spray / olive oil.

2. Beat the eggs In a large mixing bowl. Season with pepper and salt.

3. Stir in the chopped spinach, crumbled feta cheese, diced red bell pepper, and diced onion until well combined.

4. Evenly distribute the egg mixture into the greased muffin tin, filling each cup about 3/4 full.

5. Bake in the preheated oven for 20-25 minutes, or until the egg muffins are set and slightly golden on top.

6. Remove it from the oven and allow to cool for a few minutes before serving.

Cooking Time: 20-25 minutes.

Nutritional Information (per serving, based on 1 egg muffin):

- Calories: 94 kcal.

- Protein: 7g.

- Fat: 6g.

- Carbohydrates: 2g.

- Fiber: 1g.

- Sugar: 1g.

- Sodium: 165 mg.

Veggie Breakfast Wrap with Scrambled Eggs and Avocado

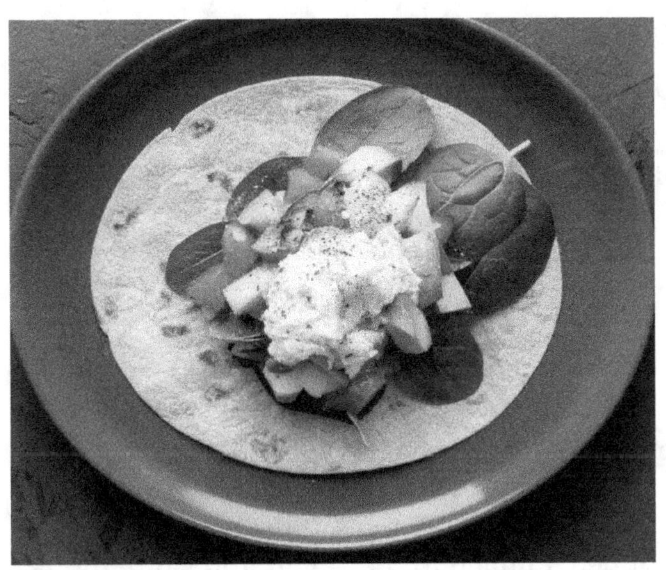

Ingredients:

- 1 whole wheat or spinach tortilla

- 2 eggs

- 1/4 cup diced bell peppers

- 1/4 cup diced tomatoes

- 1/4 cup diced onions

- 1/4 cup chopped spinach

- 1/4 avocado, sliced

- Salt and pepper to taste

- Cooking spray or olive oil.

Preparation Methods

1. In a small bowl, beat the eggs with salt and pepper.

2. Heat a non-stick skillet over medium heat and spray with cooking spray or add a small amount of olive oil.

3. Add the diced bell peppers, tomatoes, onions, and chopped spinach to the skillet and sauté for 2-3 minutes until softened.

4. Pour the whisked eggs into the skillet with the cooked vegetables.

5. Gently scramble the eggs until cooked through.

6. Warm the tortilla in a separate skillet or microwave for a few seconds until soft and pliable.

7. Place the scrambled eggs and vegetable mixture in the center of the tortilla.

8. Top with sliced avocado.

9. Fold the sides of the tortilla inward and roll it tightly to create a wrap.

Cooking Time:- Preparation: 5 minutes.

- Cooking: 5 minutes.

Nutritional Information

- Calories: 350 kcal.

- Protein: 18g.

- Carbohydrates: 25g.

- Fat: 20g.

- Fiber: 8g.

Turkey and Avocado Wrap

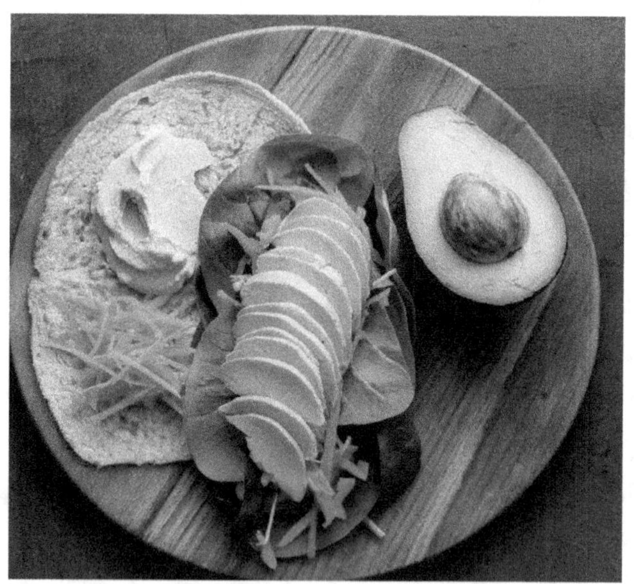

Ingredients:

- 1 whole grain wrap

- 3 ounces sliced turkey breast

- 1/4 avocado, sliced

- 1/4 cup baby spinach leaves

- 2 tablespoons shredded carrots

- 1 tablespoon hummus.

Preparation Method:

1. Lay out the whole grain wrap on a clean surface.

2. Spread hummus evenly over the wrap.

3. Layer sliced turkey breast, avocado, baby spinach leaves, and shredded carrots on top of the hummus.

4. Carefully roll up the wrap, tucking in the sides as you go.

5. Slice the wrap in half diagonally, if desired, and serve.

Nutritional Information:

- Calories: Approximately 330 kcal.

- Protein: 20g.

- Carbohydrates: 30g.

- Fat: 15g.

- Fiber: 8g.

- Sodium: 500mg.

Black Bean and Quinoa Salad

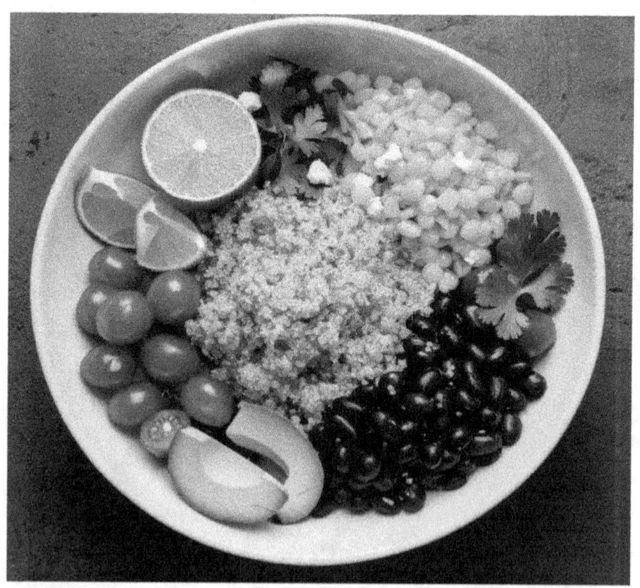

Ingredients:

- 1 cup quinoa

- 1 can (equivalent to 15 ounces) black beans, drained and washed.

- 1 cup corn kernels

- 1 red bell pepper, diced

- 1/2 cup cherry tomatoes, halved

- 1/4 cup red onion, finely chopped

- 1/4 cup fresh cilantro, chopped

- Juice of 1 lime

- 2 tablespoons extra virgin olive oil

- Salt and pepper to taste

- Optional: avocado slices, crumbled feta cheese.

Preparation:

1. Rinse quinoa under cold water. Cook quinoa according to package instructions. Fluff with a fork and let it cool once cooked.

2. In a large mixing bowl, combine cooked quinoa, black beans, corn, diced bell pepper, cherry tomatoes, red onion, and chopped cilantro.

3. In a small bowl, whisk together lime juice, olive oil, pepper, and salt.

4. Pour the dressing over the quinoa mixture and toss until everything is well coated.

5. Taste and adjust seasoning if necessary.

6. Serve immediately, or refrigerate for at least 30 minutes to allow flavors to meld.

7. Optional: Serve with avocado slices and crumbled feta cheese on top.

Cooking Time:

Cooking quinoa: 15-20 minutes

Preparation time: 10 minutes

Total time: 25-30 minutes.

Nutritional Information:

- Serving Size: 1 cup.

- Calories: **320 kcal.**

- Total Fat: **8g.**

  - Saturated Fat: **1g.**

  - Trans Fat: **0g.**

- Cholesterol: **0mg.**

- Sodium: **380mg.**

- Total Carbohydrate: **53g.**

  - Dietary Fiber: **11g.**

  - Sugars: **3g.**

- Protein: **12g.**

Tuna   Salad   Stuffed   Avocado

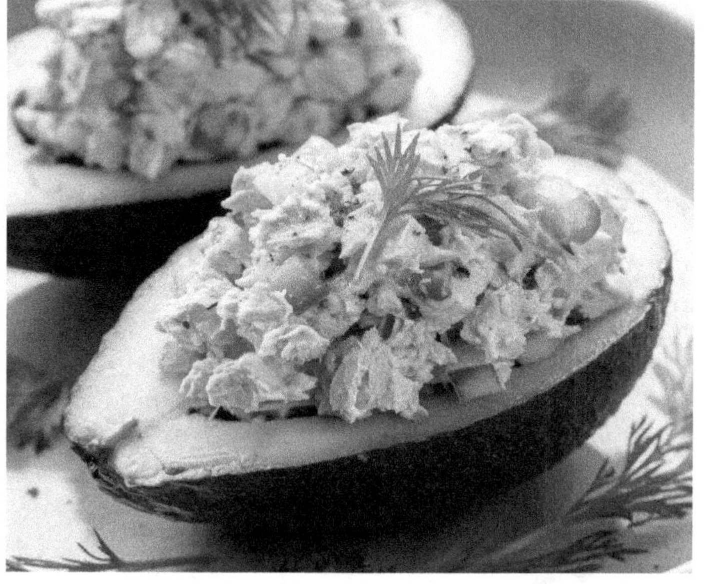

Ingredients:

- 2 ripe avocados

- 1 can (5 oz) tuna, drained

- 2 tablespoons Greek yogurt

- 1 tablespoon lemon juice

- 2 tablespoons finely chopped red onion

- 2 tablespoons finely chopped celery

- Salt and pepper, to taste

- Optional: sliced fresh parsley or dill for garnish.

Preparation Method:

1. Slice the avocados into two and remove the pits.

2. Scoop out a little bit of avocado from each half to create a larger space for the tuna salad.

3. In a mixing bowl, combine the drained tuna, Greek yogurt, lemon juice, red onion, and celery. Spice with salt and pepper to taste.

4. Spoon the tuna salad mixture into the avocado halves, dividing it evenly among them.

5. Garnish with chopped parsley or dill, if desired.

6. Serve immediately.

Cooking Time: This recipe doesn't require cooking, so the preparation time is approximately 10 minutes.

Nutritional Information:

(Per serving, based on 1 stuffed avocado half).

- Calories: 210 kcal.

- Protein: 11g.

- Fat: 14g.

- Carbohydrates: 9g.

- Fiber: 6g.

- Sugar: 1g.

- Sodium: 220mg.

Lentil Soup with Whole Grain Bread

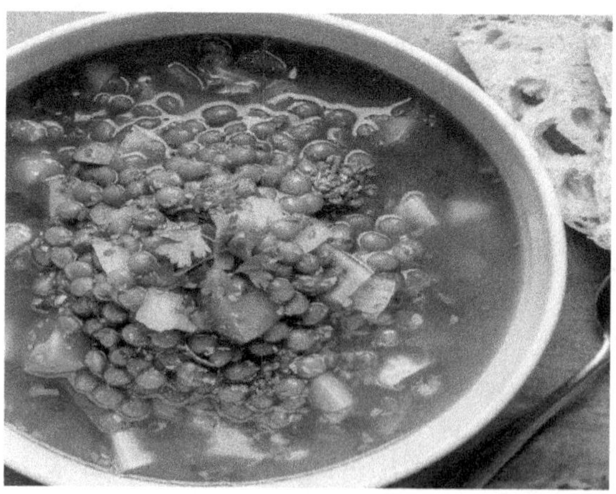

Ingredients:

- One cup dried green or brown lentils, washed and drained

- 1 onion, chopped

- 2 carrots, chopped

- 2 celery stalks, chopped

- 2 cloves garlic, minced

- 1 can (14 oz) diced tomatoes

- 4 cups vegetable broth

- 1 teaspoon ground cumin

- 1 teaspoon ground coriander

- 1/2 teaspoon smoked paprika

- Salt and pepper to taste

- Fresh parsley, chopped (for garnish)

- Whole grain bread, sliced (for serving).

Preparation:

1. In a large pot, warm up some olive oil over medium heat. Add the onion, carrots, and celery, and sauté until softened, about 5 minutes.

2. In a large pot, warm some olive oil over medium heat. Cook for another minute until they smell good.

3. Stir in the lentils, diced tomatoes, and vegetable broth. Bring the soup to a boil, then lower the heat, cover it, and let it simmer for 25-30 minutes, or until the lentils are soft.

4. Season the soup with pepper and salt to taste.

5. Ladle the soup into bowls, garnish with chopped fresh parsley, and serve with whole grain bread.

Cooking Time: Approximately 35-40 minutes.

Nutritional Information:

(Per serving, soup only)

- Calories: **250 kcal.**

- Protein: **15g.**

- Fat: **1.5g.**

- Carbohydrates: 45g

- Fiber: 15g.

- Sodium: 800mg.

Whole grain bread not included in nutritional information.

Lentil and Sweet Potato Shepherd's Pie

Ingredients:

For the Filling:

- 1 cup dry green or brown lentils.

- 2 cups vegetable broth.

- 1 tablespoon of olive oil.

- 1 onion, diced.

- 2 cloves garlic, minced.

- 2 carrots, diced.

- 2 celery stalks, diced.

- 1 teaspoon dried thyme.

- 1 teaspoon dried rosemary.

- 1 cup frozen peas.

- Salt and pepper to taste.

For the Sweet Potato Topping:

- 2 big sweet potatoes, peeled and cut into small pieces.

- 2 tablespoons butter or olive oil.

- Salt and pepper to taste.

Preparation:

1. Preheat the oven to 400°F (200°C).

2. In a large pot, combine the lentils and vegetable broth. Bring to a boil, then lower the heat and let it simmer for 20-25 minutes, or until the lentils are soft.

3. While the lentils are cooking, prepare the sweet potato topping. Place the sweet potato cubes in a pot of water and bring to a boil. Cook until the sweet potatoes are fork-tender. Strain the sweet

potatoes and place them back in the pot. Add the butter or olive oil, and mash until smooth. Spice with pepper and salt according to your liking.

4. In a big frying pan, warm the olive oil on medium heat. Put in the chopped onion and cook until it's soft, about 5 minutes. Add the minced garlic, diced carrots, and diced celery, and cook for another 5 minutes, or until the vegetables are tender.

5. Add the cooked lentils, dried thyme, dried rosemary, frozen peas, salt, and pepper to the skillet with the vegetables. Stir to combine.

6. Transfer the lentil and vegetable mixture to a baking dish. Evenly distribute the mashed sweet potatoes on top.

7. Bake in the preheated oven for 20-25 minutes, or until the sweet potato topping is lightly golden.

Cooking Time: 1 hour.

Nutritional Information:

- Serving size: 1/6 of the pie.

- Calories: Approximately 280 calories.

- Protein: Approximately 10g.

- Carbohydrates: Approximately 50g.

- Fat: Approximately 5g.

- Fiber: Approximately 12g.

Quinoa and Black Bean Stuffed Bell Peppers

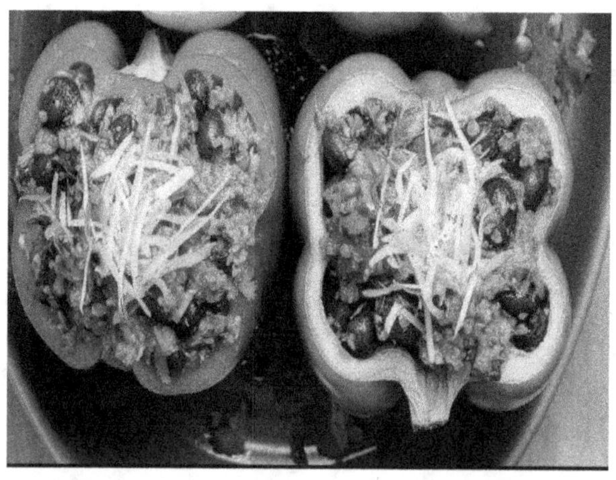

Ingredients:

- 4 large bell peppers (any color).

- 1 cup quinoa, rinsed.

- One can (15 ounces) of black beans, washed and drained.

- 1 cup corn kernels.

- 1 cup diced tomatoes.

- 1 small onion, finely chopped.

- 2 cloves garlic, minced.

- 1 teaspoon ground cumin.

- 1 teaspoon chili powder.

- 1/2 teaspoon paprika.

- Salt and pepper, to taste.

- One cup of shredded cheese (Monterey Jack, cheddar).

- Fresh cilantro, chopped (for garnish).

- Olive oil.

Preparation:

1. Preheat your oven to 375°F (190°C).

2. Cut the tops off the bell peppers and remove the membranes and the seeds. Place the bell peppers cut-side up in a baking dish and set aside.

3. In a saucepan, boil 2 cups of water. Add the quinoa, lower the heat, cover, and let it simmer for 15-20 minutes, or until the quinoa is cooked and the water is absorbed.

4. While the quinoa is cooking, heat some olive oil in a large skillet over medium heat. Add the onion and garlic and cook until they're soft, about 3-4 minutes.

5. Add the black beans, corn, diced tomatoes, cumin, chili powder, paprika, salt, and pepper to the skillet. Cook for additional 5 minutes, stirring occasionally.

6. Once the quinoa is cooked, add it to the skillet with the black bean mixture. Stir well to combine.

7. Spoon the quinoa and black bean mixture into the hollowed-out bell peppers, pressing down gently to pack the filling.

8. Sprinkle shredded cheese over the top of each stuffed pepper.

9. Cover the baking dish with aluminum foil and bake in the preheated oven for 25-30 minutes, or until the peppers are tender.

10. Remove the foil and bake for an additional 5 minutes, or until the cheese is melted and bubbly.

11. Remove from the oven and garnish with fresh cilantro before serving.

Cooking Time:

- Preparation: 15 minutes.

- Cooking: 40-45 minutes.

Nutritional Information: (per serving, based on 4 servings)

- Calories: 388 kcal.

- Protein: 17g.

- Fat: 10g.

- Carbohydrates: 62g.

- Fiber: 15g.

- Sugar: 9g.

- Sodium: 474mg.

Greek Chicken Pita Pocket with Tzatziki Sauce

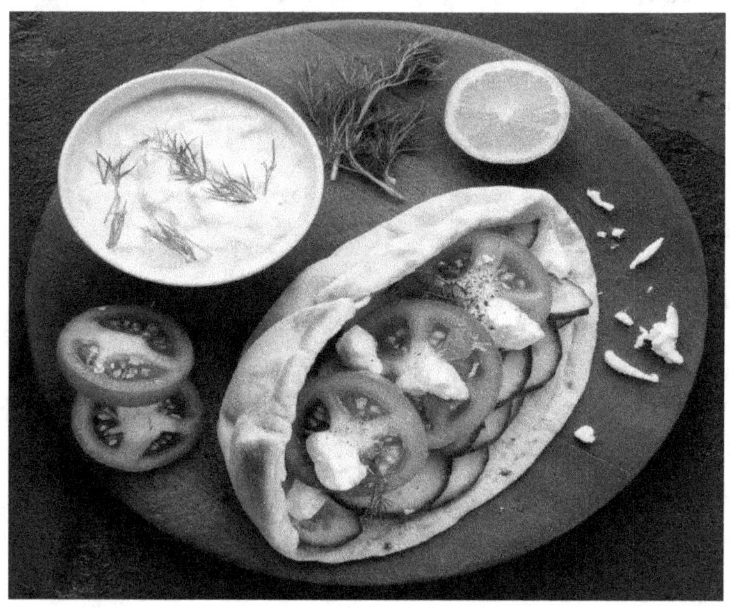

Ingredients:

For the Greek Chicken:

- 2 boneless, skinless chicken breasts.

- 1 tablespoon of olive oil.

- 2 cloves garlic, minced.

- 1 teaspoon dried oregano.

- 1 teaspoon dried thyme.

- Salt and pepper to taste.

- Juice of 1 lemon.

For the Tzatziki Sauce:

- 1 cup Greek yogurt.

- 1/2 cucumber, grated and drained.

- 1 clove garlic, minced.

- 1 tablespoon fresh dill, chopped

- 1 tablespoon lemon juice.

- Salt and pepper to taste.

For Serving:

- Whole wheat pita bread.

- Sliced tomatoes.

- Sliced red onion.

- Sliced cucumber.

- Crumbled feta cheese (optional).

- Kalamata olives (optional).

Preparation:

1. Prepare the Greek Chicken:

  - In a bowl, mix together olive oil, minced garlic, dried oregano, dried thyme, salt, pepper, and lemon juice.

  - Put the chicken breasts in the marinade, making sure they're well coated. Cover and put them in the fridge for at least 30 minutes.

- Get the grill or grill pan nice and hot over medium-high heat. Grill the chicken breasts for 6-7 minutes on each side, or until they're fully cooked. Take them off the heat and let them rest for a few minutes before slicing.

2. Prepare the Tzatziki Sauce:

- Mix Greek yogurt, grated cucumber, minced garlic, chopped dill, lemon juice, salt, and pepper in a bowl until well combined.

- Cover and put it in the fridge for at least 30 minutes so the flavors can blend together.

3. Assemble the Pita Pockets:

 - Warm the whole wheat pita bread in the oven or on the grill for a few minutes.

 - Cut the grilled chicken breasts into thin strips.

 - Open each pita pocket and spread a generous amount of tzatziki sauce inside.

 - Fill each pita pocket with sliced chicken, tomatoes, red onion, cucumber, crumbled feta cheese, and Kalamata olives if desired.

Cooking Time:

- Marinating Time: 30 minutes

- Grilling Time: 12-14 minutes

- Total Time: Approximately 45 minutes.

Nutritional Information:

- Calories: **380 kcal.**

- Protein: **32g.**

- Fat: 10g.

- Carbohydrates: 40g.

- Fiber: 6g.

- Sugar: 6g.

- Sodium: 520mg.

Chicken and Vegetable Lettuce Wraps

Ingredients:

- 1 lb (450g) ground chicken.

- 1 tablespoon of olive oil.

- 2 cloves garlic, minced.

- 1 onion, diced.

- 1 bell pepper, diced.

- 1 cup mushrooms, diced.

- 1 cup water chestnuts, chopped.

- 2 tablespoons of soy sauce.

- 1 tablespoon hoisin sauce.

- 1 teaspoon sesame oil.

- 1 teaspoon fresh ginger, minced.

- Salt and pepper to taste.

- One head of iceberg lettuce, leaves separated.

- Optional toppings: chopped green onions, cilantro, chopped peanuts.

Preparation:

1. Heat olive oil in a big frying pan over medium heat. Add minced garlic and sliced onion, cook until they start to smell good.

2. Add ground chicken to the skillet and cook until browned, breaking it apart with a spoon.

3. Add diced bell pepper, mushrooms, and water chestnuts to the skillet. Cook until vegetables are tender.

4. In a small bowl, mix together soy sauce, hoisin sauce, sesame oil, and minced ginger. Pour the

sauce over the chicken and vegetable mixture. Stir until everything is well coated.

5. Add salt and pepper to your taste.

6. To serve, spoon the chicken and vegetable mixture into individual lettuce leaves.

7. Garnish with chopped green onions, cilantro, and chopped peanuts if desired.

Cooking Time:

- Preparation: 10 minutes.

- Cooking: 15 minutes.

- Total Time: 25 minutes.

Nutritional Information:

(Per serving, assuming 4 servings).

- Calories: 250 kcal.

- Protein: 22g.

- Carbohydrates: 12g.

- Fat: 14g.

- Fiber: 4g.

- Sugar: 4g.

- Sodium: 550mg.

Zucchini Noodles with Pesto and Grilled Shrimp

Ingredients:

For the zucchini noodles:

- 4 medium zucchinis.

- 1 tablespoon of olive oil.

- Salt and pepper to taste.

For the pesto:

- 2 cups of packed fresh basil leaves.

- 1/3 cup pine nuts.

- 2 cloves garlic.

- 1/2 cup grated Parmesan cheese.

- 1/2 cup extra virgin olive oil.

- Salt and pepper to taste.

For the grilled shrimp:

- 1 pound large shrimp, peeled and deveined

- 2 tablespoons of olive oil.

- 2 cloves garlic, minced.

- 1 teaspoon paprika.

- Salt and pepper to taste.

Preparation:

1. Make the pesto:

  - Put the basil, pine nuts, garlic, and Parmesan cheese in a food processor and blend them together. Pulse until coarsely chopped.

  - With the food processor running, slowly add the olive oil until the pesto is smooth. Season with salt and pepper to taste. Set aside.

2. Prepare the zucchini noodles:

- Use a spiralizer to make zucchini noodles.

- Warm 1 tablespoon of olive oil in a big skillet over medium heat. Cook the zucchini noodles for 2-3 minutes, or until they're just tender. Season with salt and pepper to taste. Remove from heat and set aside.

3. Grill the shrimp:

 - In a bowl, toss the shrimp with 2 tablespoons of olive oil, minced garlic, paprika, salt, and pepper until evenly coated.

 - Heat a grill or frying pan on a medium high heat. Grill the shrimp for 2-3 minutes on each side until they turn pink and are fully cooked.

4. Assemble the dish:

 - In the skillet with the zucchini noodles, add the grilled shrimp and pesto. Mix everything together until it's all well combined and warmed up.

Cooking Time:

- Preparation: 15 minutes.

- Cooking: 10 minutes.

- Total: 25 minutes.

Nutritional Information:

- Servings: 4.

- Calories: Approximately 350 per serving.

- Carbohydrates: Approximately 10g per serving.

- Protein: Approximately 25g per serving.

- Fat: Approximately 25g per serving.

- Fiber: Approximately 3g per serving.

Turkey and Vegetable Stir-Fry with Brown Rice

Ingredients:

- 1 lb (450g) lean ground turkey.

- 2 cups mixed vegetables (bell peppers, broccoli, carrots, snap peas, etc.), sliced or chopped.

- 2 cloves garlic, minced.

- 1 tablespoon ginger, minced.

- 2 tablespoons of low-sodium soy sauce.

- 1 tablespoon oyster sauce (optional).

- 1 tablespoon sesame oil.

- 2 cups of cooked brown rice.

- Salt and pepper to taste.

- Green onions, chopped, for garnish (optional).

- Sesame seeds, for garnish (optional).

Preparation:

1. Heat sesame oil in a frying pan or wok over medium-high heat.

2. Add minced garlic and ginger, sauté for 1 minute until fragrant.

3. Add ground turkey to the skillet and cook until browned, breaking it apart with a spatula as it cooks.

4. Add the mixed vegetables to the skillet and cook until they are tender-crisp, about 5-7 minutes.

5. In a small bowl, mix together soy sauce and oyster sauce (if using). Pour the sauce over the turkey and vegetable mixture and stir to combine.

6. Cook for another 2-3 minutes to let the flavors mix.

7. Add salt and pepper to taste.

8. Serve the stir-fry over cooked brown rice.

9. If you like, top with chopped green onions and sesame seeds.

Cooking Time: Approximately 20 minutes.

Nutritional Information (per serving, based on 4 servings):

- Calories: 380 kcal.

- Protein: 28g.

- Carbohydrates: 40g.

- Fat: 12g.

- Fiber: 6g.

- Sugar: 3g.

Vegetable Stir-Fry with Tofu

Ingredients:

- Use one block of extra firm tofu. Press to remove excess water and cut it into cubes.

- 2 tablespoons of soy sauce.

- 1 tablespoon sesame oil.

- 1 tablespoon of olive oil.

- 2 cloves garlic, minced.

- 1 small onion, thinly sliced.

- 1 bell pepper, thinly sliced.

- 1 cup broccoli florets.

- 1 cup sliced carrots.

- 1 cup snap peas.

- Salt and pepper to taste.

- Cooked brown rice or quinoa.

- Sesame seeds and sliced green onions for garnish (optional).

Preparation:

1. Press the tofu: Place the block of tofu on a plate lined with paper towels. Put another layer of paper towels on the tofu. Then, put something heavy on top, like a heavy pan or some cans. Let the tofu press for at least 30 minutes to remove excess moisture. Once you press it, cut the tofu into cubes.

2. Marinate the tofu: In a small bowl, mix together the soy sauce and sesame oil. Toss the tofu cubes in the marinade and let them sit for 10-15 minutes.

3. Heat olive oil in a big frying pan or wok over medium-high heat. Add minced garlic and sliced onion, and cook for 2-3 minutes until softened.

4. Add the marinated tofu cubes to the skillet and cook for 5-7 minutes, stirring occasionally, until tofu is lightly browned on all sides.

5. Add the bell pepper, broccoli florets, sliced carrots, and snap peas to the skillet. Stir-fry until the vegetables are tender-crisp.

6. Spice with salt and pepper to taste.

7. Serve the vegetable stir-fry on cooked brown rice or quinoa. Top with sesame seeds and chopped green onions if you like.

Cooking Time: Approximately 20 minutes.

Nutritional Information: (Per serving, without rice or quinoa)

- Calories: **220 kcal.**

- Protein: 14g.

- Carbohydrates: 14g.

- Fat: 13g.

- Fiber: 5g.

- Sugar: 5g.

- Sodium: 500mg.

Caprese Salad with Grilled Chicken

Ingredients:

- 2 boneless, skinless chicken breasts.

- 2 large tomatoes, sliced.

- 1 ball of fresh sliced mozzarella cheese.

- Fresh basil leaves.

- Balsamic glaze.

- Salt and pepper to taste.

- Olive oil.

Preparation Method:

1. Preheat the grill to medium-high heat.

2. Season chicken breasts with salt, pepper, and a drizzle of olive oil.

3. Grill chicken for 6-7 minutes per side, or until cooked through (internal temperature of 165°F or 74°C).

4. While the chicken is cooking, arrange tomato and mozzarella slices on a plate, alternating and overlapping them.

5. Top the tomatoes and mozzarella with fresh basil leaves.

6. Once the chicken is cooked, slice it and place the slices on top of the tomato and mozzarella.

7. Drizzle with balsamic glaze and season with additional salt and pepper if desired.

Cooking Time:

- Grilling chicken: 12-14 minutes.

Nutritional Information (per serving):

- Calories: 350 kcal.

- Protein: 40g.

- Carbohydrates: 6g.

- Fat: 18g.

- Saturated Fat: 7g.

- Cholesterol: 110mg.

- Sodium: 450mg.

- Fiber: 1g.

- Sugar: 3g.

Grilled Chicken Salad

Ingredients:

- 2 boneless, skinless chicken breasts.

- 4 cups of mixed greens (spinach,lettuce , arugula etc.).

- 1 cup cherry tomatoes, halved.

- 1 cucumber, sliced.

- 1 avocado, sliced.

- 2 tablespoons balsamic vinaigrette dressing.

- Salt and pepper to taste.

Preparation:

1. Preheat the grill to medium-high heat.

2. Spice the chicken breasts with salt and pepper.

3. Grill chicken for 6-7 minutes per side, or until cooked through (internal temperature of 165°F or 75°C).

4. Remove chicken from the grill and let it rest for 5 minutes before slicing.

5. In a large bowl, toss mixed greens, cherry tomatoes, cucumber, and avocado slices.

6. Divide the salad between two plates.

7. Put sliced grilled chicken on top of each salad.

8. Drizzle with balsamic vinaigrette dressing.

9. Serve immediately.

Cooking Time:

- Total: 20-25 minutes (including prep time).

Nutritional Information (per serving):

- Calories: 380 kcal.

- Protein: 35g.

- Carbohydrates: 15g.

- Fat: 20g.

- Fiber: 8g.

- Sugar: 5g.

- Sodium: 550mg.

Vegetable and Lentil Curry with Brown Rice

Ingredients:

For the curry:

- 1 cup brown lentils, rinsed.

- 1 tablespoon of olive oil.

- 1 onion, diced.

- 3 cloves garlic, minced.

- 1 tablespoon fresh ginger, grated.

- 2 carrots, diced.

- 2 potatoes, peeled and diced.

- 1 bell pepper, diced.

- 1 zucchini, diced.

- 1 can (400g) diced tomatoes.

- 1 can (400ml) coconut milk.

- 2 tablespoons curry powder.

- 1 teaspoon turmeric.

- 1 teaspoon cumin.

- Salt and pepper to taste.

- Fresh cilantro for garnish.

For the brown rice:

- 1 cup brown rice.

- 2 cups of water.

- Pinch of salt.

Preparation:

1. Prepare Brown Rice:

- In a medium-sized pot, combine brown rice, water, and a pinch of salt.

- Heat until it boils over medium-high heat.

- Reduce heat to low, cover, and simmer for 40-45 minutes, or until rice is tender and water is absorbed.

- Use a fork to separate the grains of rice, then leave it to the side.

2. Cook Lentils:

- In a separate pot, add lentils and cover with water.

- Bring to a boil, then lower the heat and let it simmer until the lentils are soft.

- Dry any excess water and set aside.

3. Prepare Curry:

- In a big frying pan or pot, heat olive oil on medium heat.

- Add the sliced onion and cook for about 5 minutes, until it becomes see-through.

- Add minced garlic and grated ginger, and cook for another 1-2 minutes.

- Stir in diced carrots, potatoes, bell pepper, and zucchini. Cook for 5-7 minutes, until vegetables start to soften.

- Add diced tomatoes, coconut milk, curry powder, turmeric, cumin, salt, and pepper. Stir well to combine.

- Simmer uncovered for 15-20 minutes, or until vegetables are tender and the curry has thickened.

- Stir in cooked lentils and cook for another 5 minutes to heat through.

- Adjust seasoning to taste.

4. Serve:

- Serve the vegetable and lentil curry hot over brown rice.

- Garnish with fresh cilantro.

Cooking Time: Approximately 45-50 minutes.

Nutritional Information:

(Per serving, based on 4 servings).

- Calories: 450 kcal.

- Total Fat: 15g.

 - Saturated Fat: 10g.

- Cholesterol: 0mg.

- Sodium: 320mg.

- Total Carbohydrates: 67g.

 - Dietary Fiber: 15g.

 - Sugars: 10g.

- Protein: 15g.

Grilled Shrimp, Vegetable Skewers with Brown Rice

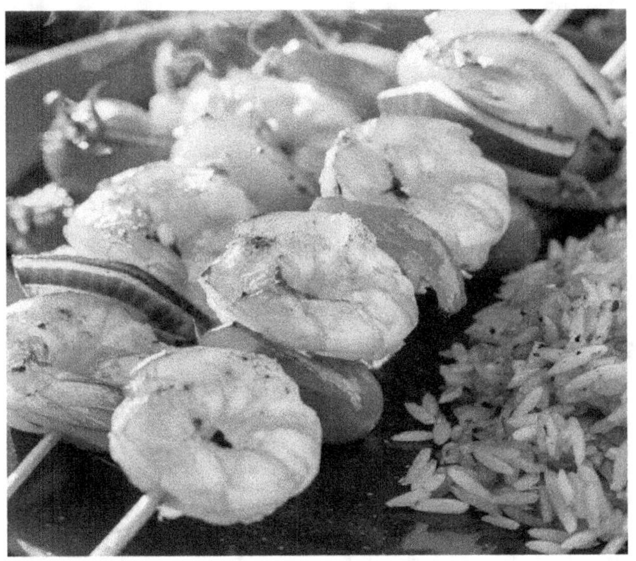

Ingredients:

For the Shrimp and Vegetable Skewers:

- 1 lb large shrimp, peeled and deveined.

- 1 red bell of pepper, sliced into pieces.

- 1 yellow bell of pepper, sliced into pieces.

- 1 red onion, cut into chunks.

- 8-10 cherry tomatoes.

- 2 tablespoons of olive oil.

- 2 cloves garlic, minced.

- 1 teaspoon paprika.

- Salt and pepper to taste.

- Wooden or metal skewers.

For the Brown Rice:

- 1 cup brown rice.

- Two cups of water or chicken broth.

- Salt to taste.

Preparation Method:

1. If you're using wooden skewers, soak them in water for at least 30 minutes so they don't burn.

2. Mix olive oil, minced garlic, paprika, salt, and pepper in a bowl. Add the shrimp and toss until

they're all coated. Let them soak in the mixture for at least 15 minutes.

3. Thread marinated shrimp, bell peppers, red onion, and cherry tomatoes onto skewers, alternating between shrimp and vegetables.

4. Preheat the grill to medium-high heat.

5. Meanwhile, rinse brown rice under cold water until the water runs clear. In a saucepan, combine rice, water or broth, and salt. Bring to a boil, then reduce the heat to low, cover, and simmer for 45 minutes or until rice is tender and water is absorbed.

6. Place the shrimp and vegetable skewers on the preheated grill. Cook for 2-3 minutes on each side, or until the shrimp is pink and opaque and the vegetables are tender and slightly charred.

7. Serve the grilled shrimp and vegetable skewers hot with brown rice.

Cooking Time:

- Marinating Time: 15 minutes

- Grilling Time: 6-8 minutes

- Total Time: Approximately 25 minutes.

Nutritional Information:

- Calories: 320 kcal.

- Protein: 25g.

- Carbohydrates: 34g.

- Fat: 10g.

- Saturated Fat: 1.5g.

- Cholesterol: 172mg.

- Sodium: 240mg.

- Fiber: 3g.

- Sugar: 3g.

Spinach, with Feta Turkey Burger and Sweet-Potato Fries

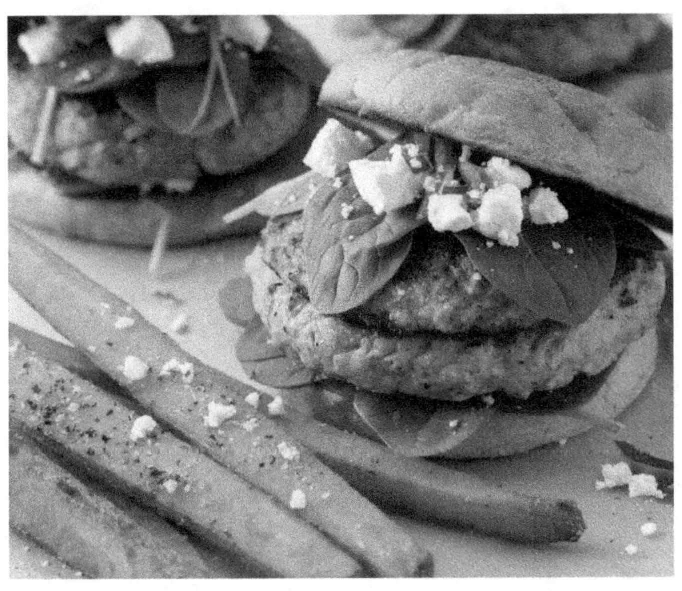

Ingredients:

For the Turkey Burgers:

- 1 lb lean ground turkey.

- 1 cup fresh spinach, chopped.

- 1/2 cup crumbled feta cheese.

- 1/4 cup finely chopped red onion.

- 2 cloves garlic, minced.

- 1 teaspoon dried oregano.

- Salt and pepper to taste.

- Whole grain burger buns.

For the Sweet Potato Fries:

- Two large sweet potatoes, cut into fry shapes.

- 2 tablespoons of olive oil.

- 1 teaspoon paprika.

- 1/2 teaspoon garlic powder.

- Salt and pepper to taste.

Preparation:

1. Preheat the oven to 425°F (220°C).

2. In a large bowl, combine the ground turkey, chopped spinach, feta cheese, red onion, minced garlic, dried oregano, salt, and pepper. Mix until well combined.

3. Divide the turkey mixture into 4 equal portions and shape each portion into a burger patty.

4. Place the sweet potato fries on a baking sheet lined with parchment paper. Sprinkle with olive oil, paprika, garlic powder, salt, and pepper. Toss to coat evenly.

5. Arrange the turkey burger patties on another baking sheet lined with parchment paper.

6. Place both baking sheets in the preheated oven. Bake the sweet potato fries for 20-25 minutes, flipping halfway through, until golden and crispy. Bake the turkey burgers for 15-20 minutes, flipping halfway through, until cooked through and no longer pink in the center.

7. Assemble the burgers by placing each turkey patty on a whole grain bun. Serve with the sweet potato fries.

Cooking Time:

- Sweet Potato Fries: 20-25 minutes.

- Turkey Burgers: 15-20 minutes.

Nutritional Information:

Turkey Burger (per serving, without bun):

- Calories: 250 kcal.

- Protein: 25g.

- Fat: 14g.

- Carbohydrates: 6g.

- Fiber: 1g.

Sweet Potato Fries (per serving):

- Calories: 150 kcal.

- Protein: 2g.

- Fat: 7g.

- Carbohydrates: 21g.

- Fiber: 4g.

Salmon Quinoa Bowl

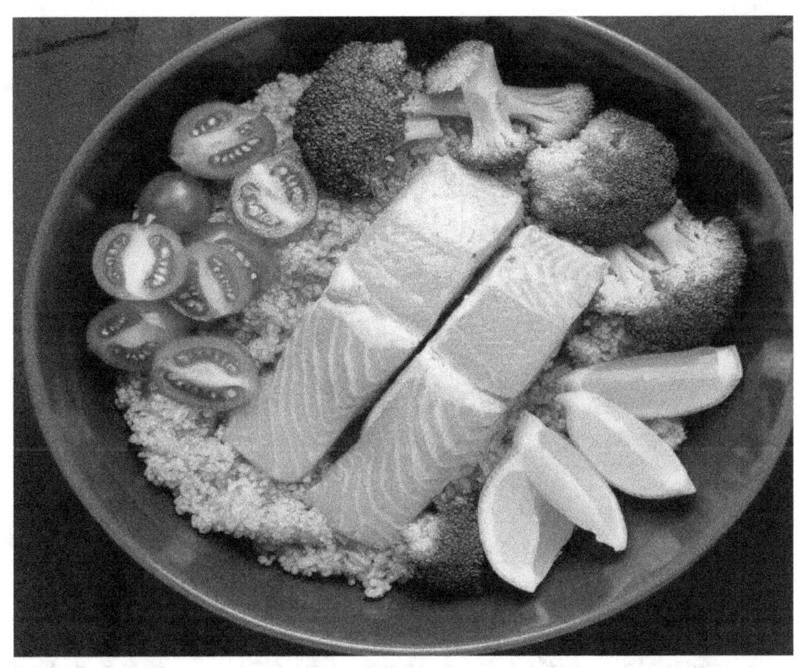

Ingredients:

- 2 salmon filets.

- 1 cup quinoa, rinsed.

- 2 cups of water or vegetable broth.

- 2 cups broccoli florets.

- 1 cup cherry tomatoes, halved.

- 1 tablespoon of olive oil.

- Salt and pepper to taste.

- Lemon wedges for serving.

Preparation:

1. Preheat the oven to 400°F (200°C).

2. Spice the salmon filets with salt, pepper, and a sprinkle of olive oil.

3. Place the salmon filets on a baking sheet lined with parchment paper.

4. In a medium saucepan, boil the water or vegetable broth. Add the quinoa, then reduce the heat to low, cover the pot, and let it simmer for about 15-20 minutes until the quinoa is cooked and the liquid is absorbed.

5. Toss the broccoli florets with olive oil, salt, and pepper, and spread them out on a separate baking sheet.

6. Place both the salmon and broccoli in the preheated oven. Roast the salmon for 12-15 minutes, or until cooked through and easily flaked

with a fork. Roast the broccoli for 15-20 minutes, or until tender and slightly browned.

7. Once the salmon and broccoli are cooked, assemble the bowls by dividing the quinoa, broccoli, and cherry tomatoes between two bowls. Garnish each bowl with a salmon fillet.

8. Serve with lemon wedges for squeezing over the salmon.

Cooking Time:

- Preparation: 10 minutes.

- Cooking: 25-30 minutes.

- Total Time: 35-40 minutes.

Nutritional Information:

- Calories: Approximately 400 calories per serving.

- Protein: Approximately 30 grams per serving.

- Fat: Approximately 15 grams per serving.

- Carbohydrates: Approximately 35 grams per serving.

- Fiber: Approximately 7 grams per serving.

Chickpea and Vegetable Buddha Bowl

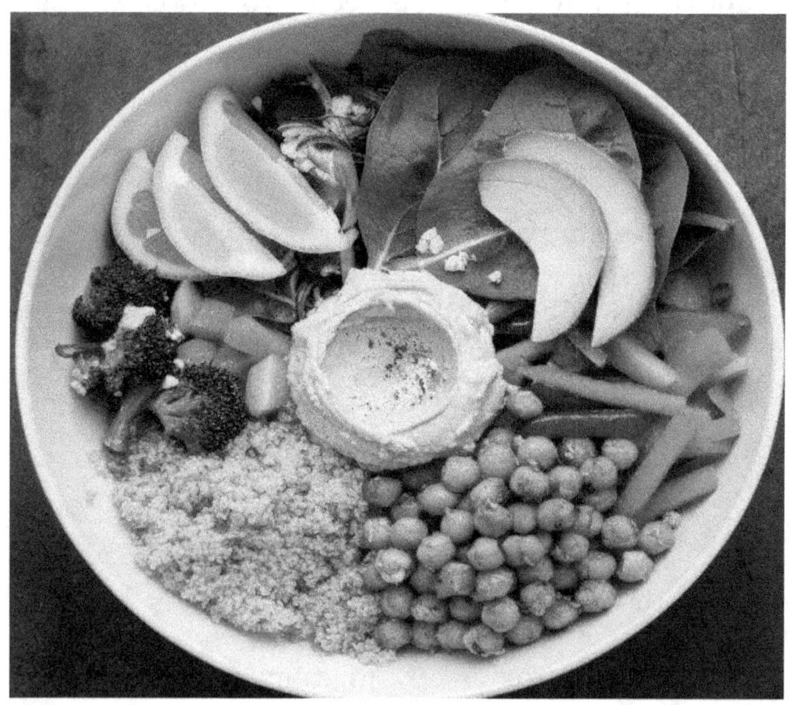

Ingredients:

For the Buddha Bowl:

- 1 cup cooked quinoa.

- 1 cup roasted chickpeas.

- 1 cup mixed vegetables (such as bell peppers, carrots, broccoli, and cauliflower).

- 2 cups of fresh spinach leaves.

- 1 avocado, sliced.

- 2 tablespoons hummus.

- 1 tablespoon of olive oil.

- Salt and pepper to taste.

- Lemon wedges for serving.

For the Lemon Tahini Dressing:

- 2 tablespoons tahini.

- 2 tablespoons of lemon juice.

- 1 tablespoon of olive oil.

- 1 clove garlic, minced.

- 2-3 tablespoons of water (to thin).

- Salt and pepper to taste.

Preparation:

1. Preheat the oven to 400°F (200°C).

2. Toss the mixed vegetables with olive oil, salt, and pepper on a baking sheet. Roast in the preheated oven for 20-25 minutes or until tender and lightly browned.

3. While the vegetables are roasting, prepare the lemon tahini dressing by whisking together tahini, lemon juice, olive oil, minced garlic, water, salt, and pepper in a small bowl. You can add more water if you want it to be thinner.

4. Assemble the Buddha bowls by dividing cooked quinoa, roasted chickpeas, roasted vegetables, fresh spinach, and sliced avocado among serving bowls.

5. Drizzle each bowl with lemon tahini dressing and hummus.

6. Serve immediately with lemon wedges on the side.

Cooking Time:

- Total: 30-35 minutes.

Nutritional Information:

- Serving Size: 1 Buddha Bowl.

- Calories: Approximately 500-550 kcal.

- Protein: Approximately 17-20 grams.

- Carbohydrates: Approximately 50-55 grams.

- Fat: Approximately 25-30 grams.

- Fiber: Approximately 15-18 grams.

Lentil and Vegetable Stew

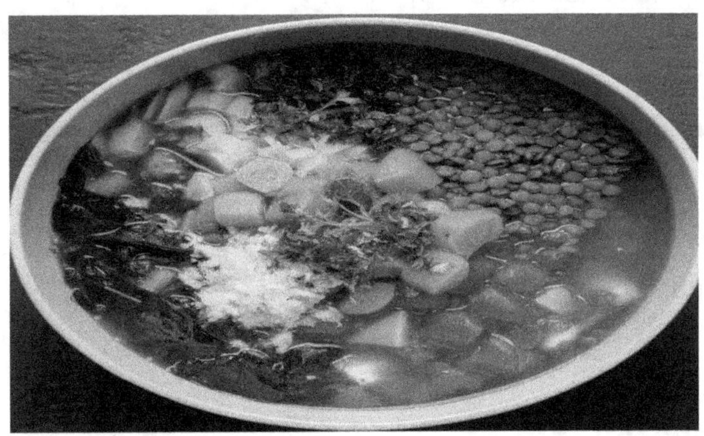

Ingredients:

- 1 cup dry green or brown lentils, rinsed and drained.

- 1 tablespoon of olive oil.

- 1 onion, diced.

- 2 carrots, diced.

- 2 celery stalks, diced.

- 2 cloves garlic, minced.

- 1 can (14 oz) diced tomatoes.

- 4 cups vegetable broth.

- 1 teaspoon dried thyme.

- 1 teaspoon dried oregano.

- Salt and pepper to taste.

- 2 cups chopped spinach or kale.

- Fresh parsley for garnish (optional).

Preparation:

1. Heat olive oil in a big pot over medium heat. Add diced onion, carrots, and celery. Cook, stirring occasionally, until vegetables are softened, about 5-7 minutes.

2. Add minced garlic and cook it for another 1-2 minutes, until fragrant.

3. Stir in lentils, diced tomatoes, vegetable broth, dried thyme, and dried oregano. Add salt and pepper to taste.

4. Allow the mixture to boil, then reduce the heat to low. Cover and simmer until the lentils are tender.

5. Stir in chopped spinach or kale and cook for an additional 5 minutes, until the greens are wilted.

6. Taste and adjust seasoning if needed. Serve hot, topped with fresh parsley if desired.

Cooking Time: 40-45 minutes.

Nutritional Information:

- Calories: **210 kcal.**

- Protein: **13g.**

- Fat: 3g.

- Carbohydrates: 36g.

- Fiber: 15g.

- Sugar: 7g.

- Sodium: 680mg.

Grilled Veggie Quesadillas with Guacamole

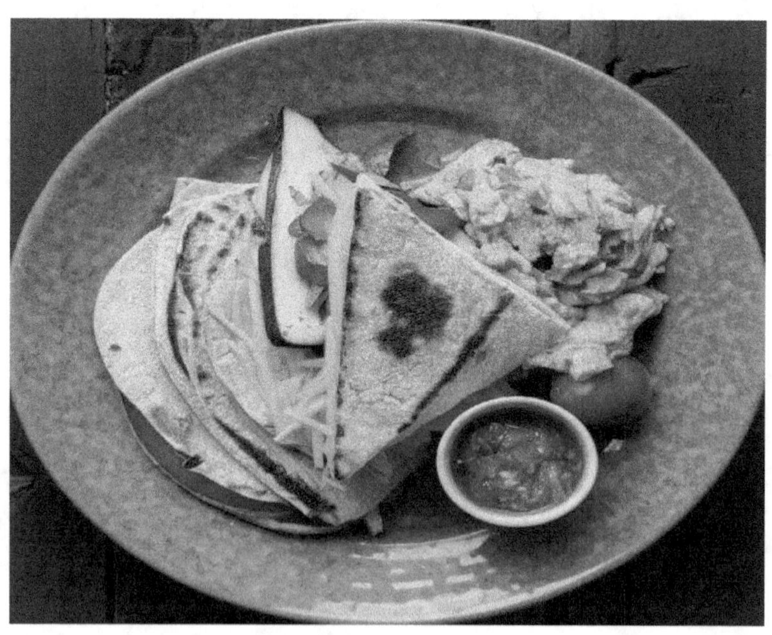

Ingredients:

- 4 large whole wheat tortillas.

- One cup of shredded cheese (cheddar, Jack, Monterey or a blend).

- 1 medium zucchini, thinly sliced.

- 1 medium bell pepper, thinly sliced.

- 1 small red onion, thinly sliced.

- 1 cup sliced mushrooms.

- 1 tablespoon of olive oil.

- Salt and pepper to taste.

- Optional: Salsa, sour cream, or Greek yogurt for serving.

- 2 ripe avocados.

- 1 small tomato, diced.

- 1/4 cup finely chopped red onion.

- 1 clove garlic, minced.

- 1 tablespoon chopped fresh cilantro.

- 1 tablespoon of lime juice.

- Salt and pepper to taste.

Preparation:

1. Prepare the Guacamole:

 - In a medium bowl, mash the avocados with a fork until smooth.

 - Stir in the diced tomato, chopped red onion, minced garlic, chopped cilantro, lime juice, salt, and pepper. Mix until well combined. Taste and adjust seasoning if necessary.

 - Cover the guacamole with plastic wrap, pressing the plastic wrap directly onto the surface to prevent browning, and refrigerate until ready to serve.

2. Prepare the Grilled Veggie Quesadillas:

 - Heat olive oil in a big frying pan over medium heat. Add the sliced zucchini, bell pepper, red onion, and mushrooms to the skillet. Season with salt and pepper. Cook, stirring occasionally, until the vegetables are tender, about 5-7 minutes. Remove from heat and set aside.

- Place a tortilla flat. Drizzle a quarter of the shredded cheese evenly over one half of the tortilla.

- Spoon a quarter of the grilled vegetables over the cheese.

- Fold the empty half of the tortilla over the filling to create a halfmoon-like shape.

- Repeat with the remaining tortillas, cheese, and grilled vegetables.

- Heat a big frying pan on a medium heat. Place the assembled quesadillas in the skillet and cook until the tortillas are golden brown and crispy and the cheese is melted, about 2-3 minutes per side.

- Remove the quesadillas from the frying pan and let them cool for a minute before slicing into wedges.

Cooking Time:

- Approximately 15-20 minutes.

Nutritional Information:

(Per serving, based on 1 quesadilla and 1/4 of the guacamole).

- Calories: 380 kcal.

- Total Fat: 22g.

 - Saturated Fat: 6g.

 - Trans Fat: 0g.

- Cholesterol: 15mg.

- Sodium: 530mg.

- Total Carbohydrates: 36g.

 - Dietary Fiber: 9g.

 - Sugars: 5g.

- Protein: 13g.

Asian-Style Chicken and Vegetable Rice Bowl

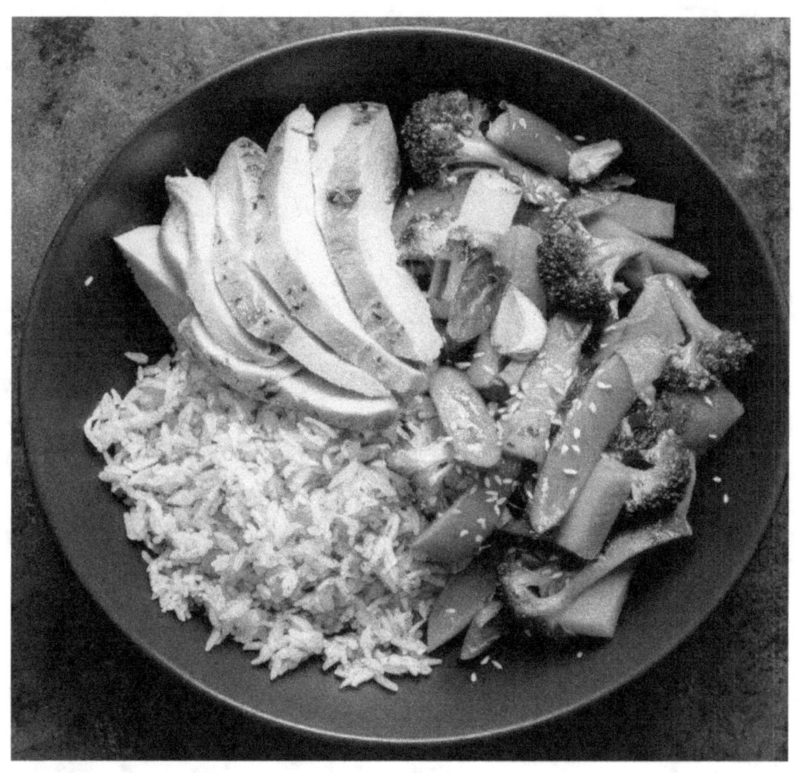

Ingredients:

For the Chicken Marinade:

- 2 chicken breasts without bones or skin, sliced thinly.

- 2 tablespoons of soy sauce.

- 1 tablespoon of honey.

- 1 tablespoon rice vinegar.

- 1 clove garlic, minced.

- 1 teaspoon grated ginger.

- 1 tablespoon sesame oil.

For the Vegetable Stir-Fry:

-2 cups of mixed vegetables (e.g bell peppers, broccoli, carrots, snap peas and carrots.)

- 1 tablespoon vegetable oil.

- 2 cloves garlic, minced.

- 1 teaspoon grated ginger.

- 2 tablespoons of soy sauce.

- 1 tablespoon oyster sauce (optional).

- Cooked brown rice, for serving.

- Sesame seeds and chopped green onions, for garnish.

Preparation:

1. Marinate the Chicken:

 - In a bowl, whisk together soy sauce, honey, rice vinegar, garlic, ginger, and sesame oil.

 - Add sliced chicken breast to the marinade and toss to coat. Cover the dish and put it in the refrigerator for at least 30 minutes.

2. Cook the Rice:

 - Prepare brown rice following the instructions on the package. Keep warm.

3. Prepare the Vegetable Stir-Fry:

 - Put vegetable oil in a big frying pan or wok over medium-high heat.

- Add minced garlic and grated ginger, and stir-fry for 30 seconds.

 - Add mixed vegetables and stir-fry for 3-4 minutes until vegetables are tender-crisp.

- Stir in soy sauce and oyster sauce (if using), cook for an additional 1-2 minutes. Remove from heat and set aside.

4. Cook the Chicken:

- In the same skillet or wok, add marinated chicken slices along with the marinade.

- Cook over medium-high heat for 5-6 minutes, stirring occasionally, until chicken is cooked through and no longer pink.

5. Assemble the Rice Bowl:

- Distribute the cooked brown rice among the serving bowls.

- Top with the vegetable stir-fry and cooked chicken slices.

- Put sliced green onions and sesame seeds on top.

Cooking Time:

- Marinating Time: 30 minutes.

- Cooking Time: 15-20 minutes.

Nutritional Information:

(Per Serving).

- Calories: 380 kcal.

- Protein: 30g.

- Carbohydrates: 45g.

- Fat: 10g.

- Fiber: 6g.

- Sugar: 8g.

- Sodium: 900mg.

Grilled Steak with Baked Sweet Potato and Asparagus

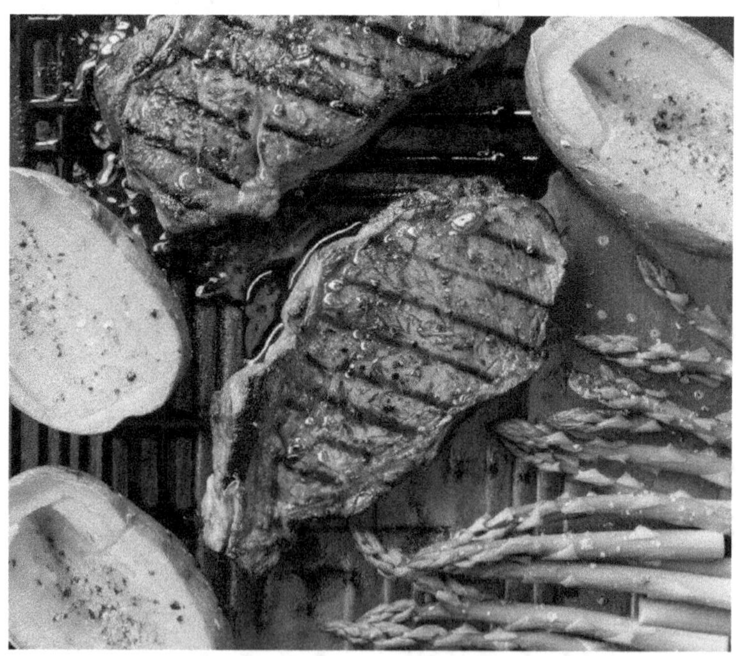

Ingredients:

For the Grilled Steak:

- 2 (6-ounce) beef steaks (such as sirloin or ribeye)

- 2 teaspoons of olive oil.

- Salt and black pepper, to taste.

For the Baked Sweet Potato:

- 2 medium sweet potatoes.

- 1 tablespoon of olive oil.

- Salt and black pepper, to taste.

For the Asparagus:

-1 bunch of asparagus with the tough ends trimmed off.

- 1 tablespoon of olive oil.

- Salt and black pepper, to taste.

Preparation Methods:

1. Grilled Steak:

- Heat the grill to medium-high heat.

 - Rub the steaks with olive oil and sprinkle them generously with salt and pepper.

 - Grill steaks for about 4-5 minutes per side for medium-rare, or until desired doneness is reached.

-Take it off the grill and let it sit for 5 minutes before serving.

2. Baked Sweet Potato:

 - Preheat the oven to 200°C.

 - Scrub sweet potatoes and dry them with a paper towel.

 - Pierce each sweet potato several times with a fork.

 - Rub sweet potatoes with olive oil and season with salt and pepper.

-Place the sweet potatoes on a baking sheet covered with parchment paper.

Bake for 45-60 minutes, or until you can easily poke it with a fork.

3. Asparagus:

- Preheat the oven to 200°C.

-Mix the asparagus with olive oil, salt, and pepper.

- Spread asparagus in a single layer on a baking sheet lined with parchment paper.

- Roast for 12-15 minutes, or until tender but still crisp.

Cooking Time:

- Grilled Steak: 10-12 minutes.

- Baked Sweet Potato: 45-60 minutes.

- Asparagus: 12-15 minutes.

Nutritional Information:

Per Serving:

- Grilled Steak:

 - Calories: **300 kcal.**

 - Protein: **30g.**

 - Fat: **18g.**

- Carbohydrates: 0g.

- **Baked Sweet Potato (1 medium):**

 - Calories: 160 kcal.

 - Protein: 2g.

 - Fat: 4g.

 - Carbohydrates: 28g.

- **Asparagus (1 cup):**

 - Calories: 27 kcal

 - Protein: 3g.

 - Fat: 1g.

 - Carbohydrates: 5g.

Shrimp and Vegetable Skewers with Quinoa

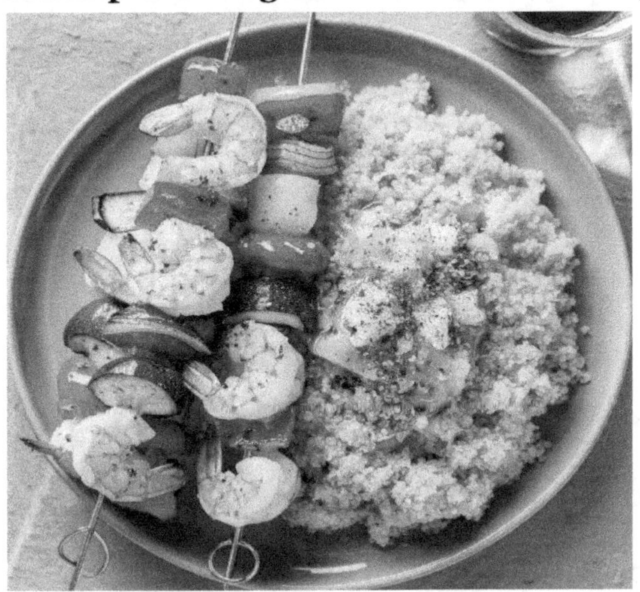

Ingredients

For the skewers

- 1 lb large shrimp, hulled and deveined.

- One red bell pepper, sliced into pieces.

- 1 unheroic bell pepper, sliced into pieces.

- 1 red onion, cut into gobbets.

- 1 zucchini, sliced into rounds.

- 1 teaspoon of olive oil painting.

- swab and pepper, to taste.

-rustic skewers, soaked for 30 twinkles in water.

For the quinoa

- 1 mug quinoa.

- Two mugs of water or vegetable broth.

- swab, to taste.

For the condiment

- 2 cloves garlic, diced.

- 2 soupspoons of olive oil painting.

- 2 soupspoons of bomb juice.

- 1 tablespoon dried oregano.

- swab and pepper, to taste.

Preparation

1. In a small coliseum, whisk together the constituents for the condiment- diced garlic, olive

oil painting, bomb juice, dried oregano, swab, and pepper. Set away.

2. In a medium saucepan, combine the quinoa, water or vegetable broth, and a pinch of swab. Bring to a pustule over medium-high heat. Reduce the heat to low, cover, and poach for 15- 20 twinkles, or until the quinoa is cooked and the liquid is absorbed. Remove from heat and let it sit, covered, for 5 twinkles. Fluff the quinoa with a chopstick and set away.

3. Preheat your frying visage over medium-high heat.

4. Thread the shrimp, bell peppers, red onion, and zucchini onto the soaked rustic skewers, interspersing between the constituents.

5. Encounter the skewers with the condiment and mizzle with olive oil painting. Season with swab and pepper.

6. Place the skewers on the preheated caff

and cook for 2- 3 twinkles per side, or until the shrimp are pink and opaque and the vegetables are tender and slightly scorched.

7. Serve the shrimp and vegetable skewers over cooked quinoa.

Cooking Time

- Prep Time 15 twinkles.

- Cook Time 10 twinkles.

-Total Time 25 twinkles.

Nutritional Information

- Servings 4.

- Calories: roughly 320 kcal per serving.

- Protein: roughly 25g per serving.

- Carbohydrates: roughly 30g per serving.

- Fat: roughly 10g per serving.

Eggplant Parmesan with Whole Wheat Pasta

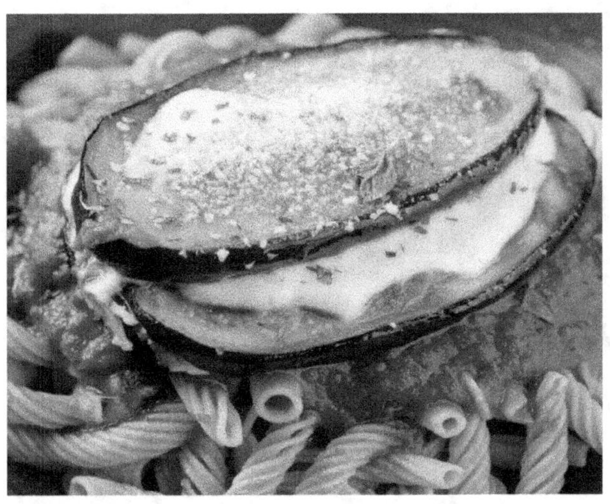

Ingredients:

For the Eggplant Parmesan:

- 2 medium eggplants, sliced into 1/4-inch rounds.

- 2 eggs.

- 1 cup whole wheat breadcrumbs.

- 1/2 cup grated Parmesan cheese.

- 1 teaspoon dried oregano.

- 1 teaspoon dried basil.

- 1/2 teaspoon garlic powder.

- Salt and pepper to taste.

- Olive oil cooking spray.

For the Assembly:

- 2 cups marinara sauce.

- 1 cup shredded mozzarella cheese.

- 1/4 cup grated Parmesan cheese.

For the Whole Wheat Pasta:

- 8 ounces whole wheat pasta.

Preparation:

1. Preheat the oven: Heat the oven to 400°F (200°C). Place parchment paper on two baking sheets and set them aside.

2. Prepare the Eggplant: In a shallow bowl, whisk the eggs. In another shallow bowl, combine the whole wheat breadcrumbs, grated Parmesan cheese, dried oregano, dried basil, garlic powder, salt, and pepper. Dip each eggplant slice into the beaten eggs, then dredge in the breadcrumb

mixture, pressing gently to adhere. Place the coated eggplant slices in a single layer on the prepared baking sheets. Spray the tops of the eggplant slices with olive oil cooking spray.

3. Bake the Eggplant: Bake in the preheated oven until the eggplant is tender and golden brown, flipping halfway through.

4. Cook the Whole Wheat Pasta: While the eggplant is baking, cook the whole wheat pasta according to the package instructions. Drain and set aside.

5. Assemble the Eggplant Parmesan: Spread 1/2 cup of marinara sauce in the bottom of a 9x13-inch baking dish. Arrange half of the baked eggplant slices on the sauce. Top the eggplant slices with 1 cup of marinara sauce, followed by half of the shredded mozzarella cheese and half of the grated Parmesan cheese. Do the same procedure with the rest of the ingredients.

6. Bake the Eggplant Parmesan: Return the baking dish to the oven and bake for an additional 20-25 minutes, or until the cheese is melted and bubbly.

7. Serve: Serve the Eggplant Parmesan hot, with the whole wheat pasta on the side.

Cooking Time:

- Preparation: 20 minutes.

- Cooking: 45 minutes.

- Total: 1 hour 5 minutes.

Nutritional Information:

- Serving Size: 1/6 of the recipe.

- Calories: **380.**

- Total Fat: **14g.**

 - Saturated Fat: **5g.**

- Cholesterol: **80mg.**

- Sodium: **810mg.**

- Total Carbohydrate: **47g.**

 - Dietary Fiber: **10g.**

 - Sugars: **9g.**

- Protein: **20g.**

Mushroom and Spinach Stuffed Chicken Breast

Ingredients:

- 4 boneless, skinless chicken breasts.

- 2 cups of fresh spinach leaves.

- 1 cup sliced mushrooms.

- 2 cloves garlic, minced.

- 1/2 cup shredded mozzarella cheese.

- Salt and pepper to taste.

- Olive oil.

Preparation:

1. Preheat your oven to 375°F (190°C).

2. Butterfly each of the chicken breast by slicing horizontally through the middle, but not all the way through, to create a pocket.

3. In a frying pan, heat a little olive oil over medium heat. Add the minced garlic and cook for 1 minute.

4. Add the sliced mushrooms to the frying pan and cook until they are soft and any liquid has evaporated, about 5-7 minutes.

5. Add fresh spinach leaves to the frying pan and cook until wilted. Spice with salt and pepper to taste.

6. Remove the skillet from the heat and let the mushroom and spinach mixture cool slightly.

7. Once cooled, stuff each chicken breast with the mushroom and spinach mixture, then sprinkle some shredded mozzarella cheese on top.

8. Secure the opening of each chicken breast with toothpicks.

9. Place the stuffed chicken breasts in a baking dish lightly coated with olive oil.

10. Bake in the preheated oven until the chicken is cooked through and the cheese is melted and bubbly.

Cooking Time: 25-30 minutes.

Nutritional Information (per serving):

- Calories: 290 kcal.

- Protein: 40g.

- Carbohydrates: 4g.

- Fat: 13g.

- Saturated Fat: 4g.

- Cholesterol: 115mg.

- Sodium: 290 mg.

- Fiber: 1g.

- Sugar: 1g.

Baked Cod with Roasted Brussels Sprouts and Cauliflower

Ingredients:

For the Baked Cod:

- 4 cod filets.

- 2 tablespoons of olive oil.

- 2 cloves garlic, minced.

- 1 tablespoon lemon juice.

- 1 teaspoon dried thyme.

- Salt and pepper to taste.

For the Roasted Brussels Sprouts and Cauliflower:

- 1 head cauliflower, cut into florets.

- 1 lb Brussels sprouts, halved.

- 2 tablespoons of olive oil.

- 2 cloves garlic, minced.

- 1 teaspoon dried thyme.

- Salt and pepper to taste.

Preparation:

1. Preheat your oven to 400°F (200°C).

2. In a small bowl, mix together the olive oil, minced garlic, lemon juice, dried thyme, salt, and pepper.

3. Place the cod filets on a baking sheet lined with parchment paper.

4. Brush the cod filets with the olive oil mixture, coating them evenly.

5. In a large bowl, toss the cauliflower florets and Brussels sprouts with olive oil, minced garlic, dried thyme, salt, and pepper until evenly coated.

6. Spread the Brussels sprouts and cauliflower on a separate baking sheet lined with parchment paper.

7. Place both baking sheets in the oven and bake for 15-20 minutes, or until the cod is cooked through and flakes easily with a fork, and the vegetables are tender and lightly browned.

Cooking Time:

- 15-20 minutes.

Nutritional Information:

Per Serving (1 cod filet with vegetables).

- Calories: **320 kcal.**

- Protein: **35g.**

- Carbohydrates: **15g.**

- Fat: **15g.**

- Fiber: **7g.**

- Sugar: **5g.**

- Sodium: **330mg.**

Beef and Broccoli Stir-Fry with Brown Rice

Ingredients:

For the stir-fry:

- 1 pound (450 grams) of beef sirloin or flank steak, sliced thinly.

- 2 cups broccoli florets.

- 1 red bell pepper, sliced.

- 1 yellow bell pepper, sliced.

- 1 onion, sliced.

- 3 cloves garlic, minced.

- 1-inch piece of ginger, grated.

- 2 tablespoons soy sauce (reduced sodium).

- 1 tablespoon oyster sauce.

- 1 tablespoon hoisin sauce.

- 1 tablespoon cornstarch.

- 2 tablespoons vegetable oil.

- Salt and pepper to taste.

- Cooked brown rice, for serving.

Preparation:

1. In a small bowl, whisk together soy sauce, oyster sauce, hoisin sauce, and cornstarch. Set aside.

2. Heat 1 tablespoon of vegetable oil in a large frying pan over medium-high heat.

3. Add sliced beef to the frying pan and stir-fry until browned, about 2-3 minutes. Remove beef from the frying pan and keep aside.

4. Add the remaining tablespoon of vegetable oil to the skillet.

5. Add minced garlic and grated ginger to the skillet and sauté for 1 minute.

6. Add sliced onion, bell peppers, and broccoli florets to the skillet. Stir-fry it for 3-4 minutes until vegetables the are tender-crisp.

7. Put back the cooked beef to the skillet.

8. Pour the sauce on the beef and vegetables in the skillet. Stir well to coat everything evenly.

9. Cook for an additional 2-3 minutes until the sauce has thickened.

10. Spice with salt and pepper to taste.

11. Serve the beef and broccoli stir-fry hot over cooked brown rice.

Cooking Time:

- Preparation Time: 15 minutes.

- Cooking Time: 15 minutes.

- Total Time: 30 minutes.

Nutritional Information:

- Serving Size: 1/4 of the recipe (not including brown rice).

- Calories: Approximately 320 kcal.

- Protein: Approximately 25g.

- Carbohydrates: Approximately 14g.

- Fat: Approximately 18g.

- Fiber: Approximately 4g.

- Sodium: Approximately 700mg.

Thai Basil Chicken with Brown Rice

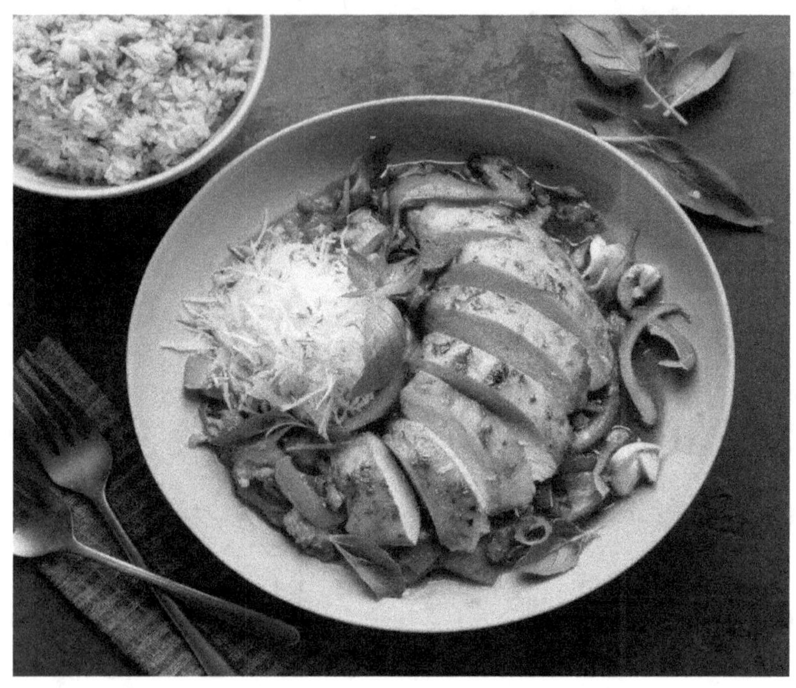

Ingredients:

For the Thai Basil Chicken:

- 1 lb (450g) boneless, chicken breasts without skin, thinly sliced.

- 2 tablespoons of soy sauce.

- 1 tablespoon oyster sauce.

- 1 tablespoon fish sauce.

- 1 tablespoon brown sugar.

- 2 tablespoons vegetable oil.

- 4 cloves garlic, minced.

- One red chili, thinly sliced.

- 1 bell pepper, thinly sliced.

- 1 onion, thinly sliced.

- 1 cup fresh basil leaves.

For the Brown Rice:

- 1 cup brown rice.

- 2 cups of water.

Preparation Method:

1. Cook Brown Rice:

  - Wash the brown rice under cold water until the water runs clear.

  - In a medium sauce-pan, boil 2 cups of water .

- Put the washed brown rice to the boiling water.

- Reduce the heat to low, cover, and simmer until the rice is tender and the water is absorbed.

- Once cooked, fluff the rice with a fork and keep aside.

2. Prepare Thai Basil Chicken:

- In a small bowl, whisk together soy sauce, oyster sauce, fish sauce, and brown sugar. Set aside.

- Heat vegetable oil in a big frying pan over medium-high heat.

- Add minced garlic and sliced chili (if using) to the skillet and cook for 1 minute until fragrant.

- Add the sliced chicken breasts to the frying pan and stir-fry for 3-4 minutes until cooked through.

- Push the chicken to one side of the frying pan and add sliced bell pepper and onion. Cook for an additional two to three minutes until the vegetables are tender.

- Pour the sauce over the chicken and vegetables. Stir well to combine.

- Add fresh basil leaves to the frying pan and toss until the basil is wilted.

- Remove from heat.

Cooking Time:

- Total cooking time: Approximately 30 minutes.

- Prep time: 10 minutes.

- Cook time: 20 minutes.

Nutritional Information:

Thai Basil Chicken (per serving, without rice):

- Calories: **250 kcal.**

- Protein: **25g.**

- Fat: **11g.**

- Carbohydrates: **12g.**

- Fiber: **2g.**

- Sugar: **6g.**

- Sodium: **1050mg.**

Brown Rice (per serving):

- Calories: **216 kcal.**

- Protein: 5g.

- Fat: 1g.

- Carbohydrates: 45g.

- Fiber: 4g.

- Sugar: 0g.

- Sodium: **6mg.**

Teriyaki Tofu Stir-Fry with Brown Rice

Ingredients:
For the Teriyaki Sauce:
- 1/4 cup low-sodium soy sauce.
- One tablespoons of honey (or maple syrup).
- 1 tablespoon rice vinegar.
- 1 teaspoon sesame oil.
- 2 cloves garlic, minced.
- 1 teaspoon grated ginger.
- 1 tablespoon cornstarch.

- 2 tablespoons of water.
For the Stir-Fry:
- 14oz or 400g of firm tofu, pressed and cubed.
- 2 cups mixed vegetables (e.g bell peppers, carrots, broccoli, snap peas).
- 2 tablespoons vegetable oil.
- 2 cups of cooked brown rice.
- Sesame seeds, for garnish (optional).
- Sliced green onions, for garnish (optional).

Preparation:
1. In a small bowl, whisk together soy sauce, honey (or maple syrup), rice vinegar, sesame oil, minced garlic, and grated ginger to make the teriyaki sauce.
2. In another small bowl, mix cornstarch and water to make a slurry.
3. In a big frying pan or wok, heat 1 tablespoon of vegetable oil over medium-high heat. Add cubed tofu and cook until golden brown on all sides, about 5-7 minutes. Remove tofu from the frying pan and set aside.
4. In the same frying pan, add the remaining tablespoon of vegetable oil. Add mixed vegetables and stir-fry for 3-4 minutes, until they are crisp-tender.

5. Return the tofu to the frying pan and pour the teriyaki sauce over the tofu and vegetables. Stir to coat everything in the sauce.

6. Add the cornstarch slurry to the skillet and stir well. Cook for another two to three minutes, until the sauce has thickened.

7. Serve the teriyaki tofu stir-fry with cooked brown rice. Top with sesame seeds and sliced green onions, (optional).

Cooking Time:
- Preparation: 15 minutes.
- Cooking: 15 minutes.
- Total Time: 30 minutes.

Nutritional Information:
- Servings: 4.
- Calories per serving: Approximately 350 kcal.
- Protein: 15g.
- Carbohydrates: 45g.
- Fat: 12g.
- Fiber: 6g.
- Sugar: 10g.
- Sodium: 650mg.

Spaghetti Squash with Turkey Bolognese Sauce

Ingredients:

For the Spaghetti Squash:

- 1 medium spaghetti squash.

- Olive oil.

- Salt and pepper.

For the Turkey Bolognese Sauce:

- 1 lb (450g) lean ground turkey.

- 1 onion, finely chopped.

- 2 cloves garlic, minced.

- 1 carrot, finely chopped.

- 1 celery stalk, finely chopped.

- 1 can (14 ounces / 400 grams) of crushed tomatoes.

- 2 tablespoons tomato paste.

- 1 teaspoon dried oregano.

- 1 teaspoon dried basil.

- Salt and pepper, to taste.

- Fresh basil leaves, for garnish (optional).

- Grated Parmesan cheese, for serving (optional).

Preparation:

1. Preheat the oven to 400°F (200°C).

2. Cut the spaghetti squash lengthwise and remove the seeds.

3. Drizzle the inside of the squash halves with olive oil and season with salt and pepper.

4. Put the squash halves, cut side down, on a baking sheet lined with parchment paper.

5. Roast in the heated oven for 40-45 minutes, (or until the squash is tender and easily pierced with a fork).

6. While the squash is roasting, prepare the turkey bolognese sauce.

7. In a large skillet, heat some olive oil over medium heat. Add the sliced onion, garlic, celery, and carrot, and sauté until softened, about 5 minutes.

8. Add the ground turkey to the skillet and cook until browned, breaking it up with a spoon as it cooks.

9. Stir in the crushed tomatoes, tomato paste, dried oregano, and dried basil. Spice with salt and pepper to your liking.

10. Simmer the sauce for 15-20 minutes, stirring occasionally, until it thickens slightly.

11. Once the spaghetti squash is done, use a fork to scrape the flesh into spaghetti-like strands.

12. Serve the spaghetti squash topped with the turkey bolognese sauce.

13. Garnish with fresh basil leaves and grated Parmesan cheese, if desired.

Cooking Time:

- Spaghetti Squash: 40-45 minutes.

- Turkey Bolognese Sauce: 30 minutes.

Nutritional Information:

- Serving Size: 1/4 of the recipe.

- Calories: approximately 300 kcal.

- Protein: approximately 25g.

- Carbohydrates: approximately 30g.

- Fat: approximately 10g.

- Fiber: approximately 7g.

Ratatouille with Grilled Chicken

Ingredients:

For Ratatouille:
- 1 small eggplant, diced.
- 1 zucchini, diced.
- 1 yellow squash, diced.
- 1 red bell pepper, diced.
- 1 onion, diced.
- 2 cloves garlic, minced.
- 2 cups sliced tomatoes (canned or fresh).
- 2 tablespoons tomato paste.

- 1 teaspoon dried thyme.
- 1 teaspoon dried oregano.
- Salt and pepper to taste.
- 2 tablespoons of olive oil.

For Grilled Chicken:
- 2 boneless, skinless chicken breasts.
- Salt and pepper to taste.
- 1 tablespoon of olive oil.

Preparation:
1. Preheat the grill to medium-high heat.

2. In a big frying pan, heat two tablespoons of olive oil over medium heat. Add the diced onion and minced garlic, and cook until softened, about 3-4 minutes.

3. Add the diced eggplant, zucchini, yellow squash, and red bell pepper to the skillet. Cook and stir the vegetables now and then until they are soft, which should take about 10 minutes.

4. Stir in the diced tomatoes, tomato paste, dried thyme, dried oregano, salt, and pepper. Simmer the ratatouille mixture for another 10-15 minutes,

stirring occasionally, until the flavors have melded together and the mixture has thickened slightly.

5. While the ratatouille is simmering, season the chicken breasts with salt, pepper, and olive oil.

6. Grill the chicken breasts for 6-7 minutes per side, or until they are cooked through and have nice grill marks.

7. Serve the grilled chicken alongside the ratatouille.

Cooking Time:
- Ratatouille: Approximately 25-30 minutes.
- Grilled Chicken: Approximately 12-14 minutes.

Nutritional Information:
- Ratatouille (per serving):
 - Calories: **120 kcal.**
 - Protein: **2g.**
 - Fat: **7g.**
 - Carbohydrates: **14g.**
 - Fiber: **5g.**
 - Sugar: **7g.**

- Grilled Chicken (per serving):

- Calories: 180 kcal.
- Protein: 25g.
- Fat: 9g.
- Carbohydrates: 0g.
- Fiber: 0g.
- Sugar: 0g.

Grilled Pork Tenderloin with Roasted Root Vegetables

Ingredients:

For the Pork Tenderloin:

- 1 pork tenderloin (about 1 lb).

- 2 cloves garlic, minced.

- 2 tablespoons of olive oil.

- 1 tablespoon balsamic vinegar.

- 1 teaspoon dried thyme.

- Salt and pepper to taste.

For the Roasted Root Vegetables:

- 2 medium carrots, peel them and cut them into 1-inch pieces.

- Two medium parsnips, peeled and cut into 1-inch pieces.

- Two medium sweet potatoes, peeled and cut into 1-inch pieces.

- One medium-sized red onion, cut into wedges.

- 2 tablespoons of olive oil.

- 1 teaspoon dried rosemary.

- Salt and pepper to taste.

Preparation:

1. Preheat the grill to medium-high heat.

2. In a small bowl, whisk together minced garlic, olive oil, balsamic vinegar, dried thyme, salt, and pepper.

3. Place the pork tenderloin in a shallow dish and pour the marinade over it. Turn to coat the tenderloin evenly. Leave it to soak for at least 30

minutes, or you can keep it in the fridge for up to 4 hours.

4. Preheat the oven to 400°F (200°C).

5. In a large bowl, toss together the carrots, parsnips, sweet potatoes, and red onion with olive oil, dried rosemary, salt, and pepper until evenly coated.

6. Spread the vegetables in a single layer on a baking sheet.

7. Roast the vegetables in the preheated oven for 25-30 minutes, or until tender and lightly browned, stirring halfway through.

8. While the vegetables are roasting, grill the marinated pork tenderloin on the preheated grill, turning occasionally, until the internal temperature reaches 145°F (63°C), about 15-20 minutes.

9. Remove the pork tenderloin from the grill and let it rest for 5 minutes before slicing.

Cooking Time:

- Marinating time: 30 minutes to 4 hours.

- Grill time: 15-20 minutes.

- Roast time: 25-30 minutes.

Nutritional Information:

Pork Tenderloin (per serving):

- Calories: **200 kcal.**

- Protein: **25g.**

- Carbohydrates: **2g.**

- Fat: **10g.**

- Fiber: **0g.**

- Sugar: **1g.**

- Sodium: **80mg.**

 Roasted Root Vegetables (per serving):

- Calories: **150 kcal.**

- Protein: **2g.**

- Carbohydrates: **20g.**

- Fat: **7g.**

Lemon Garlic Shrimp with Spinach and Whole Grain Couscous

Ingredients:

For the Lemon Garlic Shrimp:

- One pound large shrimp, peeled and deveined.

- 4 cloves garlic, minced.

- Zest of 1 lemon.

- Juice of 1 lemon.

- 2 tablespoons of olive oil.

- Salt and pepper to taste.

- 2 tablespoons chopped fresh parsley.

For the Spinach:

- 4 cups of fresh spinach leaves.

- 1 tablespoon of olive oil.

- 2 cloves garlic, minced.

- Salt and pepper to taste.

For the Whole Grain Couscous:

- 1 cup whole grain couscous.

- 1 1/4 cups of water.

- Salt to taste.

- 1 tablespoon of olive oil.

Preparation:

1. Prepare the Lemon Garlic Shrimp:

  - In a bowl, combine the shrimp with minced garlic, lemon zest, lemon juice, olive oil, salt, and pepper. Toss to coat the shrimp evenly.

  - Let the shrimp marinate for at least fifteen minutes.

- Heat a big frying-pan on a medium-high heat. Add the marinated shrimp to the frying pan and cook for 2-3 minutes on each side, until pink and cooked through.

- Sprinkle chopped parsley over the shrimp before serving.

2. Prepare the Spinach:

- Heat olive oil in a separate frying pan on a medium heat.

- Add minced garlic and sauté for one minute until fragrant.

- Add fresh spinach leaves to the frying pan and sauté for 2-3 minutes, until wilted.

- Add salt and pepper to taste.

3. Prepare the Whole Grain Couscous:

- In a medium sauce-pan, allow the water to boil.

- Stir in whole grain couscous and salt. Cover, remove from heat, and let stand for 5 minutes.

- Fluff couscous with a fork, drizzle with olive oil, and stir to combine.

Cooking Time:

- Preparation Time: 10 minutes.

- Cooking Time: 15 minutes.

- Total Time: 25 minutes.

Nutritional Information:

- Lemon Garlic Shrimp (per serving, based on 4 servings):

 - Calories: **224 kcal.**

 - Protein: **23g.**

 - Fat: **9g.**

 - Carbohydrates: **11g.**

 - Fiber: **1g.**

 - Sugar: **0g.**

- Sodium: **214 mg.**

- Spinach (per serving, based on 4 servings):

- Calories: **43 kcal.**

- Protein: **2g.**

- Fat: **3g.**

- Carbohydrates: **4g.**

- Fiber: **2g.**

- Sugar: **0g.**

- Sodium: **48mg.**

- Whole Grain Couscous (per serving, based on 4 servings):

- Calories: **169 kcal.**

- Protein: **6g.**

- Fat: **3g.**

- Carbohydrates: **32g.**

- Fiber: **4g.**

- Sugar: 0g.

- Sodium: 0mg.

Vegetable and Chickpea Curry

Ingredients:

- 1 tablespoon of olive oil.

- 1 onion, chopped.

- 2 cloves garlic, minced.

- 1 tablespoon fresh ginger, grated.

- 2 teaspoons curry powder.

- 1 teaspoon ground cumin.

- 1 teaspoon ground coriander.

- 1/2 teaspoon turmeric.

- 1/4 teaspoon cayenne pepper (optional).

- 1 can (14 oz) chickpeas, drained and washed.

- 1 can (14 ounces) diced tomatoes.

- 1 can (14 ounces) coconut milk.

- 2 cups mixed vegetables (such as carrots, bell peppers, and spinach), chopped.

- Salt and pepper to taste.

- Fresh cilantro, chopped (for garnish).

- Cooked brown rice, for serving.

Preparation:

1. Heat olive oil in a big frying pan over medium heat.

2. Add chopped onion and cook until softened, about 5 minutes.

3. Add minced garlic and grated ginger, and cook for another 2 minutes.

4. Stir in curry powder, cumin, coriander, turmeric, and cayenne pepper (if using), and cook for 1 minute, until fragrant.

5. Add chickpeas, diced tomatoes, coconut milk, and mixed vegetables to the skillet. Stir well to combine.

6. Let the mixture start bubbling, then reduce the heat. Cover and let it simmer gently for 15-20 minutes, stirring occasionally, until the vegetables are tender.

7. Spice with salt and pepper to taste.

8. Serve the vegetable and chickpea curry over cooked brown rice, garnished with chopped fresh cilantro.

Cooking Time: Approximately 25 minutes.

Nutritional Information:

- Serving Size: 1/4 of the recipe (excluding rice).

- Calories: **280.**

- Total Fat: **15g.**

  - Saturated Fat: **10g.**

- Cholesterol: **0mg.**

- Sodium: **350mg.**

- Total Carbohydrate: **30g.**

  - Dietary Fiber: **7g.**

- Total Sugars: **8g.**

- Protein: **8g.**

Cauliflower Crust Pizza with Chicken and Vegetables

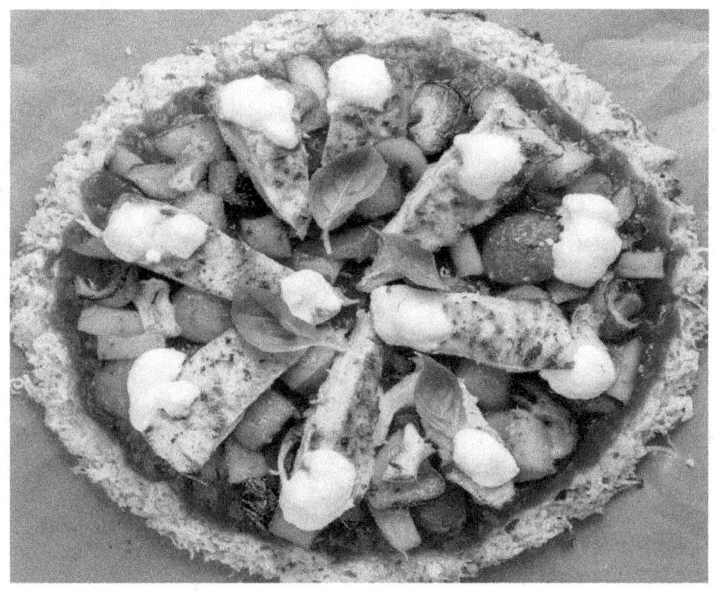

Ingredients:

For the cauliflower crust:

- 1 medium cauliflower, grated into small pieces (about 4 cups).

- 1/2 cup shredded mozzarella cheese.

- 1/4 cup grated Parmesan cheese.

- 1/2 teaspoon dried oregano.

- 1/2 teaspoon dried basil.

- 1/2 teaspoon garlic powder.

- 1/4 teaspoon salt.

- 1/4 teaspoon black pepper.

- 1 large egg.

For the pizza toppings:

- 1/2 cup marinara sauce.

- 1 cup cooked chicken breast, diced.

- 1 cup mixed vegetables (bell peppers, onions, mushrooms etc.), sliced.

- 1/2 cup shredded mozzarella cheese.

- Fresh basil leaves, for garnish (optional).

Preparation:

1. Preheat the oven to 425°F (220°C). Line a baking sheet with parchment paper and put aside.

2. To make the cauliflower crust, place the riced cauliflower in a microwave-safe bowl and microwave on high for 4-5 minutes, or until softened. Allow to cool slightly.

3. Once cooled, transfer the cauliflower to a clean kitchen towel and wring out as much moisture as possible.

4. In a mixing bowl, combine the cauliflower, shredded mozzarella cheese, Parmesan cheese, dried oregano, dried basil, garlic powder, salt, black pepper, and egg. Mix until well combined.

5. Transfer the cauliflower mixture to the prepared baking sheet and spread it out into a thin, round crust shape, about 1/4 inch thick.

6. Bake the cauliflower crust in the preheated oven for 15-20 minutes, or until golden brown and firm to the touch.

7. Once the crust is baked, remove it from the oven and spread the marinara sauce evenly over the crust.

8. Top the sauce with diced chicken breast, mixed vegetables, and shredded mozzarella cheese.

9. Put the pizza back in the oven and bake for another 10-15 minutes, or until the cheese is melted and bubbling.

10. Take the pizza out of the oven and let it cool for a few minutes before cutting it.

11. Garnish with fresh basil leaves, if desired, before serving.

Cooking Time:

- Preparation: 15 minutes.

- Cooking: 35-40 minutes.

- Total Time: 50-55 minutes.

Nutritional Information:

- Calories: **280 kcal.**

- Carbohydrates: **12g.**

- Fiber: 4g.

- Sugar: 4g.

- Fat: 15g.

- Saturated Fat: 6g.

- Protein: 25g.

- Sodium: 670mg.

Turkey and Vegetable Chili

Ingredients:

- 1 lb lean ground turkey.

- 1 tablespoon of olive oil.

- 1 onion, diced.

- 2 cloves garlic, minced.

- 1 bell pepper, diced.

- 2 carrots, diced.

- 2 stalks of celery, diced.

- 1 can (15 ounces) diced tomatoes.

- 1 can (15 ounces) of kidney beans, drained and rinsed.

- 1 can (15 oz) black beans, washed and drained.

- 1 cup corn kernels (fresh, frozen, or canned).

- 2 cups of chicken or vegetable broth with low sodium.

- 2 tablespoons of chili powder.

- 1 teaspoon ground cumin.

- 1 teaspoon paprika.

- Salt and pepper to taste.

- Optional toppings: shredded cheese, sliced green onions, Greek yogurt or sour cream, chopped cilantro, avocado slices.

Preparation:

1. Heat olive oil in a big pot over medium heat. Add the diced onion, garlic, bell pepper, carrots, and celery. Cook, stirring occasionally, until the

vegetables are softened, about five to seven minutes.

2. Add the ground turkey to the pot. Break it apart with a spoon and cook until browned, about 5 minutes.

3. Stir in the diced tomatoes, kidney beans, black beans, corn, chicken or vegetable broth, chili powder, cumin, paprika, salt, and pepper.

4. Bring the chili to a boil, then reduce the heat to low and let it simmer, uncovered, for about 30 minutes, stirring occasionally.

5. Taste and adjust seasoning as needed. Serve hot with the toppings you like.

Cooking Time: Approximately 45 minutes.

Nutritional Information (per serving, without toppings):

- Calories: **320 kcal.**

- Protein: **27g.**

- Fat: **8g.**

- Carbohydrates: 34g.

- Fiber: 9g.

- Sugar: 6g.

- Sodium: 580mg.

Grilled Chicken with Roasted Vegetables

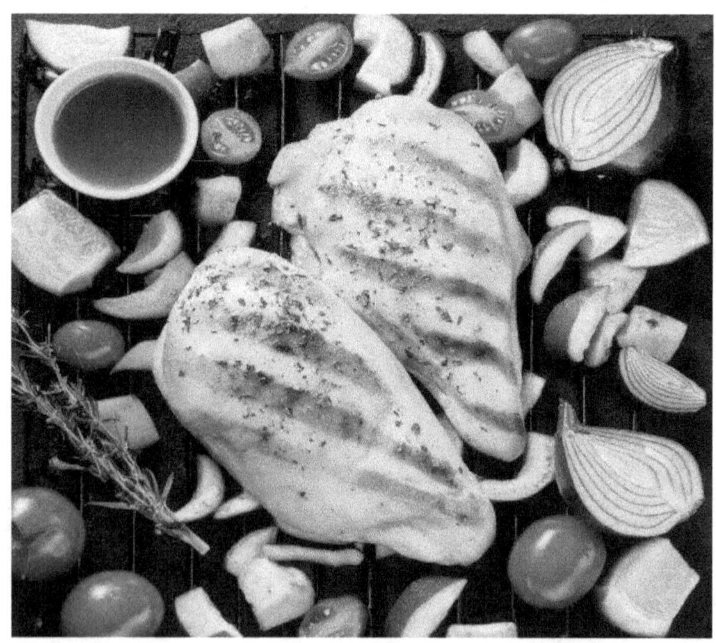

Ingredients:

- 2 boneless, skinless chicken breasts

- 2 cups mixed vegetables (such as bell peppers, zucchini, red onion, and cherry tomatoes).

- 2 tablespoons of olive oil.

- Salt and pepper, to taste.

- 1 teaspoon of dried herbs like thyme, rosemary, or Italian seasoning.

Preparation Method:

1. Preheat your grill to medium-high heat.

2. Season the chicken breasts with salt, pepper, and dried herbs.

3. Mix the mixed vegetables with olive oil, salt, and pepper.

4. Grill the chicken breasts for 6-7 minutes per side, or until they reach an internal temperature of 165°F (75°C) and are cooked through.

5. While the chicken is grilling, place the mixed vegetables on a baking sheet in a single layer.

6. Roast the vegetables in the oven at 400°F (200°C) for 15-20 minutes, or until they are tender and slightly caramelized.

Cooking Time:

- Grilling the chicken: 12-14 minutes.

- Roasting the vegetables: 15-20 minutes.

Nutritional Information:

- Calories: Approximately 300 calories per serving.

- Protein: Approximately 30 grams per serving.

- Carbohydrates: Approximately 10 grams per serving.

- Fat: Approximately 15 grams per serving.

- Fiber: Approximately 4 grams per serving.

Chicken Caesar Salad with Whole Grain Croutons

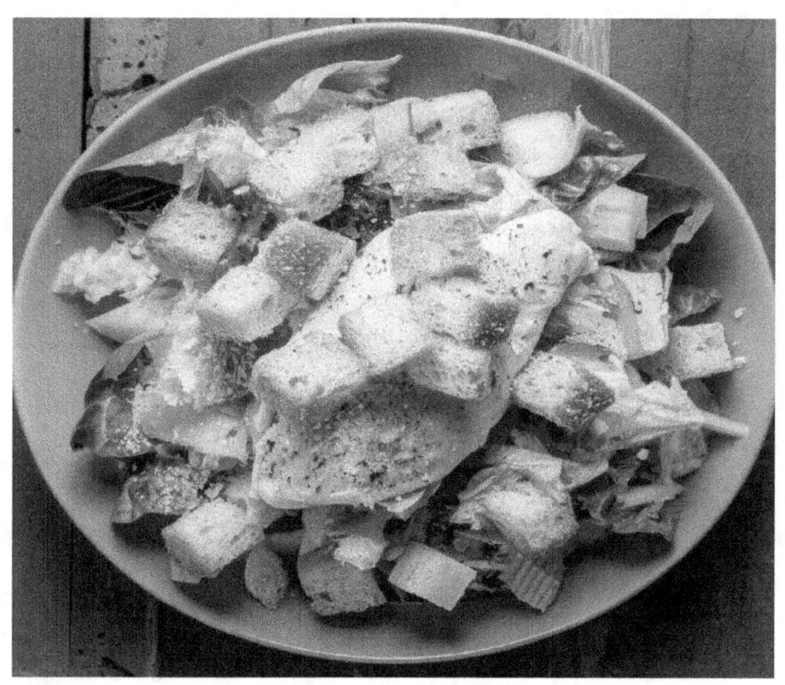

Ingredients:

For the Salad:

- 2 boneless, skinless chicken breasts.

- 1 tablespoon of olive oil.

- Salt and black pepper to taste.

- 1 head romaine lettuce, chopped.

- 1/4 cup grated Parmesan cheese.

- Whole grain croutons (see recipe below).

- 1/4 cup Greek yogurt.

- 2 tablespoons mayonnaise.

- 2 tablespoons grated Parmesan cheese.

- 1 tablespoon lemon juice.

- 1 teaspoon Dijon mustard.

- 1 clove garlic, minced.

- Salt and black pepper to taste.

For the Whole Grain Croutons:

- 2 cups whole grain bread, cut into cubes.

- 1 tablespoon of olive oil.

- 1/2 teaspoon garlic powder.

- Salt and black pepper to taste.

Preparation:

1. Prepare the Chicken:

 - Heat the grill or grill pan over medium-high heat before using.

 - Rub the chicken breasts with olive oil and season with salt and black pepper.

 - Grill the chicken for 6-8 minutes on each side, or until it's cooked through.

Take it off the heat and let it rest for 5 minutes before slicing.

2. Prepare the Dressing:

 - In a small bowl, whisk together the Greek yogurt, mayonnaise, Parmesan cheese, lemon juice, Dijon mustard, minced garlic, salt, and black pepper until well combined. Set aside.

3. Prepare the Whole Grain Croutons:

 - Heat the oven to 375°F (190°C).

 - In a large bowl, toss the whole grain bread cubes with olive oil, garlic powder, salt, and black pepper until evenly coated.

- Spread the bread cubes in one layer on a baking sheet.

- Bake for 10-12 minutes until they turn golden brown and crispy.

- Remove them from the oven and let them cool.

4. Assemble the Salad:

 - In a large bowl, combine the chopped romaine lettuce, grated Parmesan cheese, and sliced grilled chicken.

 - Add the whole grain croutons.

 - Drizzle with the prepared Caesar dressing and toss until everything is well coated.

Cooking Time:

- Grilling the chicken: 12-16 minutes.

- Making the croutons: 10-12 minutes.

- Assembling the salad: 10 minutes.

Nutritional Information:

- Calories: **320** kcal.

- Protein: 30g.

- Fat: 14g.

- Carbohydrates: 20g.

- Fiber: 5g.

- Sugar: 4g.

- Sodium: 480mg.

Stuffed Bell Peppers

Ingredients:

- 4 large bell peppers (any color).

- 1 cup cooked quinoa.

- One lb lean beef or turkey.

- 1 cup diced tomatoes (fresh).

- 1 cup cooked black beans.

- 1 cup corn kernels (or canned).

- 1 small onion, diced.

- 2 cloves garlic, minced.

- 1 teaspoon chili powder.

- 1 teaspoon cumin.

- Salt and pepper to taste.

- 1 cup shredded cheese (mozzarella, cheddar, or a blend).

- Chopped fresh cilantro.

Preparation:

1. Heat your oven to 375°F (190°C).

2. Cut the tops off the bell peppers and remove the seeds and insides.

3. In a large skillet, cook the ground beef or turkey over medium heat until brown. Remove any extra fat.

4. Add the diced onion and minced garlic to the skillet and cook for another 2-3 minutes until softened.

5. Mix in the cooked quinoa, diced tomatoes, black beans, corn, chili powder, cumin, salt, and pepper. Cook for an extra 5 minutes to blend the flavors.

6. Fill each bell pepper with the quinoa and meat mixture, pressing down gently to pack it in.

7. Place the stuffed bell peppers in a baking dish.

8. Cover the baking dish with aluminum foil and bake in the preheated oven for 25-30 minutes, or until the peppers are soft.

9. Remove the foil, sprinkle the shredded cheese over the tops of the peppers, and return them to the oven for an additional 5 minutes, or until the cheese is melted and bubbly.

10. Remove from the oven and garnish with chopped cilantro or parsley if desired before serving.

Cooking Time:

- Prep Time: 20 minutes.

- Cook Time: 35-40 minutes.

- Total Time: 55-60 minutes.

Nutritional Information:

- Servings: 4.

- Calories: Approximately 400 calories per serving.

- Protein: Approximately 25 grams per serving.

- Carbohydrates: Approximately 40 grams per serving.

- Fat: Approximately 15 grams per serving.

- Fiber: Approximately 9 grams per serving.

Quinoa-Stuffed Acorn Squash

Ingredients:

- 1 cup dry green or brown lentils, rinse, and drain it.

- 1 tablespoon of olive oil.

- 1 onion, diced.

- 2 carrots, diced.

- 2 celery stalks, diced.

- 2 cloves garlic, minced.

- 1 can (14 oz) diced tomatoes.

- 4 cups vegetable broth.

- 1 teaspoon dried thyme.

- 1 teaspoon dried oregano.

- Salt and pepper to taste.

- 2 cups chopped spinach or kale.

- Fresh parsley for garnish (optional).

Preparation:

1. Heat olive oil in a big pot over medium heat. Add diced onion, carrots, and celery. Cook, stirring occasionally, until vegetables are softened, about 5-7 minutes.

2. Add minced garlic and cook for another 1-2 minutes until it smells fragrant.

3. Stir in lentils, diced tomatoes, vegetable broth, dried thyme, and dried oregano. Season with salt and pepper to taste.

4. Bring the mixture to a boil, then turn the heat down to low. Cover and simmer until the lentils are tender.

5. Stir in chopped spinach or kale and cook for an additional 5 minutes, until the greens are wilted.

6. Taste and adjust seasoning if needed. Serve hot, topped with fresh parsley if desired.

Cooking Time: 40-45 minutes.

Nutritional Information(per serving, for six servings):

- Calories: **210 kcal.**

- Protein: **13g.**

- Fat: **3g.**

- Carbohydrates: **36g.**

- Fiber: **15g.**

- Sugar: **7g.**

- Sodium: 680mg.

Turkey Meatballs with Zucchini Noodles

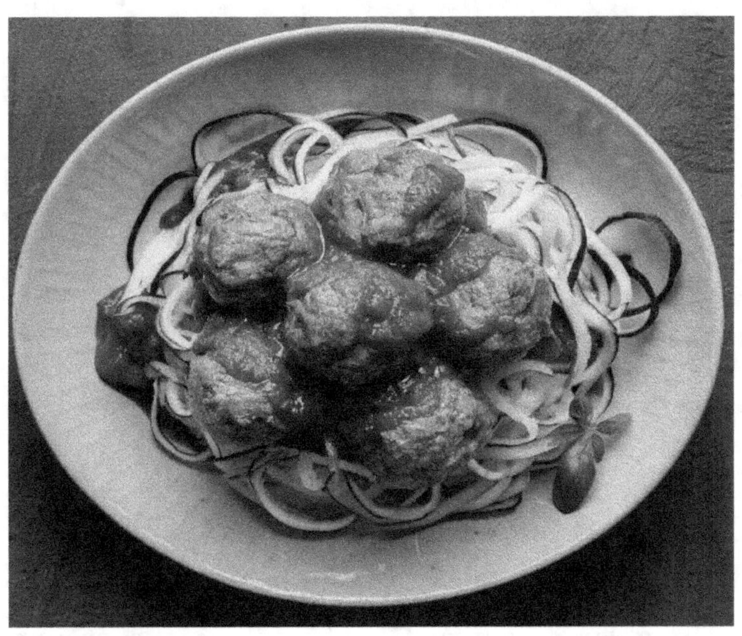

Ingredients:

- 1 lb lean ground turkey.

- 1/4 cup whole wheat breadcrumbs.

- 1/4 cup grated Parmesan cheese.

- 1 large egg.

- 2 cloves garlic, minced.

- 1 teaspoon dried oregano.

- 1 teaspoon dried basil.

- Salt and pepper to taste.

- 4 medium zucchini, spiralized into noodles.

- 2 cups marinara sauce.

- Fresh basil leaves for garnish (optional).

Preparation:

1. Preheat the oven to 375°F (190°C). Cover a baking sheet with parchment paper or lightly grease it with olive oil.

2. In a large mixing bowl, combine the ground turkey, breadcrumbs, Parmesan cheese, egg, minced garlic, oregano, basil, salt, and pepper. Mix until well combined.

3. Shape the turkey mixture into meatballs, about 1 inch in diameter, and place them on the prepared baking sheet.

4. Bake the meatballs in the preheated oven for 20-25 minutes or until cooked through and browned on the outside.

5. While the meatballs are baking, spiralize the zucchini into noodles using a spiralizer.

6. Heat the marinara sauce in a large skillet over medium heat. Once the meatballs are done, add them to the skillet with the marinara sauce and let them simmer for a few minutes.

7. In a separate skillet, heat a little olive oil over medium heat. Add the zucchini noodles and sauté for two to three minutes until just tender.

8. Serve the turkey meatballs and marinara sauce over the zucchini noodles. Top with fresh basil leaves if you want.

Cooking Time:

- Prep Time: 15 minutes.

- Cook Time: 20-25 minutes.

- Total Time: 35-40 minutes.

Nutritional Information:

- Serving Size: 4 meatballs with zucchini noodles and sauce.

- Calories: 320 kcal.

- Total Fat: 12g.

 - Saturated Fat: 3g.

- Cholesterol: 130mg.

- Sodium: 620mg.

- Total Carbohydrates: 19g.

 - Dietary Fiber: 4g.

 - Sugars: 8g.

- Protein: 33g.

Baked Salmon with Quinoa and Steamed Broccoli

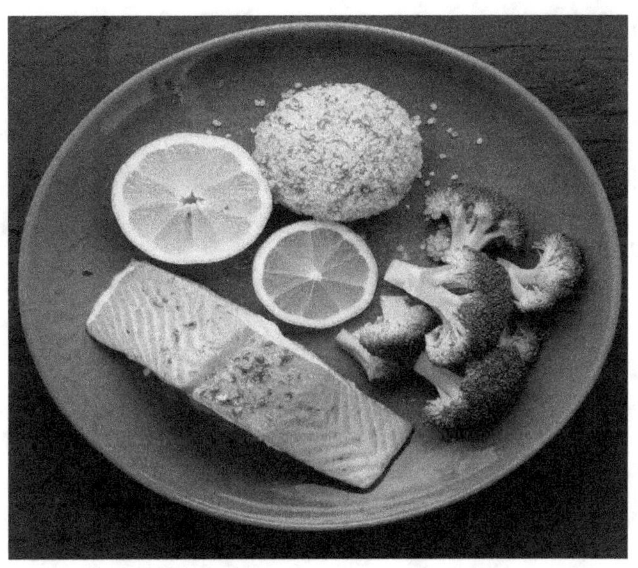

Ingredients:

For Baked Salmon:

- 4 salmon filets.

- 2 tablespoons of olive oil.

- 2 cloves garlic, minced.

- 1 teaspoon dried oregano.

- 1 teaspoon dried thyme.

- Salt and pepper to taste.

- Lemon slices for garnish (optional).

For Quinoa:

- 1 cup quinoa.

- Two cups of water/vegetable broth.

- Salt to taste.

For Steamed Broccoli:

- Slice 2 broccoli heads into small pieces.

- Salt to taste.

Preparation Methods:

1. Preheat your oven to 375°F (190°C).

2. Rinse the quinoa under cold water until the water runs clear.

3. In a medium saucepan, boil 2 cups of water or vegetable broth. Add quinoa and salt, reduce heat to low, cover, and simmer for 15-20 minutes, or until quinoa is cooked and water is absorbed. Fluff with a fork and put aside.

4. While the quinoa is cooking, prepare the salmon. Put salmon filets on a baking sheet lined with parchment paper.

5. In a small bowl, mix together olive oil, minced garlic, dried oregano, dried thyme, salt, and pepper.

6. Brush the olive oil mixture over the salmon filets.

7. Bake salmon in the preheated oven for 12-15 minutes, or until the salmon is cooked through and flakes easily with a fork.

8. While the salmon is baking, steam the broccoli. Put broccoli florets in a steamer basket over boiling water. Cover and steam for 5-7 minutes, or until broccoli is tender but still crisp.

9. Once everything is cooked, serve the baked salmon with cooked quinoa and steamed broccoli. Garnish with lemon slices if desired.

Cooking Time:

- Baked Salmon: **12-15 minutes.**

- Quinoa: **15-20 minutes.**

- Steamed Broccoli: **5-7 minutes.**

Nutritional Information:

Per serving:

- Calories: 450 kcal.

- Protein: 38g.

- Carbohydrates: 30g.

- Fat: 20g.

- Fiber: 6g- Sodium: 450mg.

CHAPTER 8

CARDIOVASCULAR TRAINING FOR ENDOMORPHS

Cardiovascular training, also known as cardio, is an essential component of any fitness routine, especially for endomorphs who may have a slower metabolism and find it harder to lose weight. Here are some cardio training pointers specifically for endomorphs:

1. Include a Variety of Cardio Exercises

- Mix it up with different types of cardio exercises, such as walking, jogging, cycling, swimming, dancing, and aerobic classes.

- Try high-intensity interval training (HIIT) workouts, which involve short bursts of intense exercise followed by periods of rest or lower-intensity exercise. HIIT can enhance metabolism and burn more calories in a short period of time.

2. Focus on Duration and Intensity

   - Aim for at least 150 minutes of moderate-intensity cardio exercise per week or 75 minutes of vigorous-intensity cardio exercise a week.

 - Slowly increase the duration and intensity of your exercise as your fitness level improves.

3. Monitor Your Heart Rate

 - Use a heart rate monitor to track your heart rate during cardio workouts.

 - Aim to reach your target heart rate zone, which is typically 50-85% of your maximum heart rate, depending on your fitness goals and fitness level.

Strength Training Strategies

Strength training is another important component of a well-rounded fitness routine, especially for endomorphs, who may struggle to build and maintain muscle mass. Here are some strength training strategies for endomorphs:

1. Focus on Compound Exercises

- Compound exercises target multiple muscle groups at once and are more effective for building strength and muscle mass.
- Compound exercises, such as squats, deadlifts, lunges, bench presses, pull-ups, and rows, are examples of effective strength-training movements.

2. Use Progressive Overload

- Gradually increase the weight, reps, or sets of your strength training exercises over time to continually challenge your muscles and promote muscle growth.
- Aim to work each major muscle group 2-3 times per week with a day of rest in between.

3. Include Both Upper and Lower Body Exercises

- Balance your strength training routine by including exercises that target both the upper and lower body.
- This helps to improve overall muscle tone and balance and prevent muscle imbalances.

4. Incorporate Bodyweight Exercises

- Bodyweight exercises are an excellent way to increase strength and muscle mass without requiring any equipment.
- Include exercises like push-ups, squats, lunges, and planks in your routine.

Flexibility and Mobility Work

Flexibility and mobility are often overlooked but are essential for overall health and fitness, especially for endomorphs, who may be prone to carrying excess weight and have a higher risk of injury. Here are some flexibility and mobility exercises to incorporate into your routine:

1. Stretching

- Include both static and dynamic stretches to improve flexibility and range of motion.
- Focus on stretching all major muscle groups, including the chest, back, shoulders, arms, legs, and hips.

2. Foam Rolling

- Utilize a foam roller to relieve tight muscles and enhance flexibility.

- Foam rolling can help reduce muscle soreness, improve circulation, and increase flexibility.

3. Mobility Drills
 - Incorporate mobility drills and exercises that focus on improving joint mobility and stability.
 - Include exercises like hip circles, shoulder circles, leg swings, and arm circles in your warm-up routine.

4. Yoga and Pilates
 - Consider adding yoga or Pilates classes to your routine to improve flexibility, balance, and core strength.
 - Both yoga and Pilates are excellent for improving posture, reducing stress, and promoting overall well-being.

By incorporating cardiovascular training, strength training, flexibility, and mobility work into fitness routine, endomorphs can optimize their metabolism, build muscle, and improve overall health and fitness.

CHAPTER 9

OVERCOMING CHALLENGES AND PLATEAUS

Experiencing a weight loss plateau is common, especially for endomorphs who may have a slower metabolism and find it harder to lose weight. However, there are several strategies you can use to overcome a weight loss plateau and continue making progress towards your goals:

1. Review Your Diet and Exercise Routine
- Take a closer look at your diet and exercise habits to identify any areas where you may be slipping up or becoming complacent.

 - Are you still following your meal plan and exercise routine as consistently as before? Are there areas where you need to improve?

2. Adjust Your Calorie Intake
 - As you lose weight, your body requires a little calories to sustain your new weight. If you've hit a plateau, try reducing your calorie intake slightly to kickstart weight loss again.

- Be careful not to drastically reduce your calorie intake, as this can slow down your metabolism and make it harder to lose weight in the long run.

3. Change Up Your Exercise Routine

- If you've been doing the same workouts for a while, your body may have adapted to the routine, leading to a plateau.
- Try incorporating new exercises, increasing the intensity or duration of your workouts, or trying different types of cardio or strength training exercises to challenge your body in new ways.

4. Focus on Non-Scale Victories

- Sometimes the scale doesn't budge, even when you're making progress in other areas.
- Focus on other signs of progress, such as how your clothes fit, improvements in strength and endurance, or changes in body composition.

5. Stay Consistent and Patient

- Always remember that weight loss takes time, and it's normal to hit plateaus along the way.
- Stay consistent with your healthy habits, be patient, and trust the process, the results will come.

Managing Emotional Eating

It can be an uphill struggle to lose weight when you're dealing with emotional eating, especially when you're stressed, feeling anxious, or sad. Here are some strategies to help you manage emotional eating:

1. Identify Triggers
-Be conscious of the scenerios, events or emotions that trigger emotional eating for you.
 - Keeping a food journal can help you identify patterns and triggers.

2. Find Alternative Coping Strategies
 - Instead of turning to food for comfort, find other ways to cope with your emotions, such as going for a walk, talking to a friend, practicing deep breathing or meditation, or engaging in a hobby or activity you enjoy.

3. Practice Mindful Eating
 - Slow down and pay attention to what you're eating. Eat mindfully, savoring each bite, and paying attention to hunger and fullness cues.
 - Avoid eating in front of the TV or computer, as this can lead to mindless eating.

4. **Stock Up on Healthy Snacks**
 - Keep healthy snacks on hand so that when you do feel the urge to eat, you have nutritious options available.
 - Choose snacks that are high in protein and fiber, such as nuts, Greek yogurt, fruits, and vegetables.

5. **Seek Support**
 - If you find yourself contending with emotional eating, do not delay to reach out for support. Talk to some friend, a therapist or family member who can offer advice and support.

CHAPTER 10

SUPPLEMENTS FOR ENDOMORPHS

While a healthy diet and regular exercise are the most important factors for weight loss and supporting metabolism, some supplements may help endomorphs reach their goals more effectively. Here are some supplements that may support weight loss and metabolism:

1. Protein Powder
 - Protein is essential for building and repairing muscle, and it can also help increase feelings of fullness and support weight loss.
 - Whey protein, casein protein, and plant-based protein powders are popular options that can be added to smoothies, oatmeal, or yogurt.

2. Green Tea Extract
- Green tea contains catechins, antioxidants that can potentially increase metabolism and aid in fat loss.

- Green tea extract supplements are available in pill or powder form and can be taken as a supplement or added to beverages.

3. Caffeine

- Caffeine is a natural stimulant that can help increase energy levels, boost metabolism, and improve exercise performance.
- Caffeine supplements are available in pill or powder form, or you can simply enjoy a cup of coffee or green tea.

4. Conjugated Linoleic Acid (CLA)

- CLA, a fatty acid, has been shown to potentially decrease body fat and enhance lean muscle mass.
- CLA supplements are available in pill form and are often derived from safflower oil or sunflower oil.

5. Fiber Supplements

- Fiber aids to promote feelings of fullness, regulate blood sugar levels, and also support digestive health.
- Fiber supplements such as psyllium husk or glucomannan can be taken in pill or powder form.

6. **Fish Oil**
 - Fish oil is rich in omega-3 fatty acids, which have been shown to reduce inflammation, improve heart health, and support weight loss.
 - Fish oil supplements come in either pill or liquid form.

It's important to note that while these supplements may support weight loss and metabolism, they are not a substitute for a healthy diet and regular exercise. It's always best to focus on getting nutrients from whole foods whenever possible and use supplements to fill in any gaps in your diet.

Vitamins and Minerals for Endomorphs

Endomorphs may have unique nutritional needs, and certain vitamins and minerals can play a role in supporting metabolism and overall health. Here are some vitamins and minerals that endomorphs should pay particular attention to:

1. **Vitamin D**
 - Vitamin D plays a role in regulating metabolism and may help support weight loss.

- Endomorphs may be at a higher risk of vitamin D deficiency, especially if they live in northern climates or spend limited time outdoors.

2. Calcium

- Calcium is essential for bone health and may also help support weight loss by promoting fat breakdown.

- Calcium-rich foods such as dairy products, leafy green vegetables, and fortified foods are beneficial for your health.

3. **Magnesium**

- Magnesium is involved in over 300 biochemical reactions in the body, including metabolism and energy production.

- Foods rich in magnesium includes nuts, seeds, whole grains, and leafy green vegetables.

4. **Iron**

- Iron is essential for transporting oxygen throughout the body and plays a role in metabolism and energy production.

- Endomorphs, especially women, may be at a higher risk of iron deficiency.

5. B vitamins (B6, B12, folate)

- B vitamins are important for energy metabolism and may help support weight loss and overall health.
- Foods rich in B vitamins include meat, fish, poultry, eggs, dairy products, legumes, and leafy green vegetables.

6. Chromium

- Chromium is a mineral that may help regulate blood sugar levels and support weight loss.
- Chromium-rich foods include broccoli, barley, oats, green beans, and tomatoes.

While it's possible to get these vitamins and minerals from food sources, some endomorphs may benefit from taking a multivitamin or specific supplements to ensure they're meeting their nutritional needs. However, it's essential to talk to a healthcare professional before starting any new supplements to ensure they're safe and appropriate for you.

CHAPTER 11

LIFESTYLE STRATEGIES FOR SUCCESS

Managing stress is crucial for overall health and well-being, especially for endomorphs who may be more prone to emotional eating and weight gain during times of stress. Below are some of the helpful stress management techniques:

1. Regular Exercise
- Physical activity is an effective stress reliever and mood enhancer. Strive for a minimum of 30 minutes of moderate-intensity exercise on most days of the week.
- Find activities you enjoy, whether it's walking, jogging, cycling, swimming, dancing, or yoga.

2. Deep Breathing Exercises
- Deep breathing exercises can help activate the body's relaxation response and reduce stress levels.
- Try the 4-7-8 breathing technique: Inhale deeply through your nose for a count of 4, hold your breath

for a count of 7, and then exhale slowly through your mouth for a count of 8.

3. Mindfulness and Meditation
 - Mindfulness and meditation techniques can help quiet the mind, reduce stress, and improve overall well-being.
 - Practice mindfulness by focusing on the present moment, paying attention to your thoughts and feelings without judgment.
 - There are numerous guided meditation apps and online videos to assist you in getting started.

4. Yoga and Tai Chi
 - Yoga and tai chi are gentle forms of exercise that combine movement, breath, and mindfulness.
 - Both practices can help reduce stress, improve flexibility and balance, and promote overall well-being.

5. Get Outside
 - Spending quality time in nature can have a calming effect on the mind and body.
 - Take a stroll in the park, go for a hike, or just relax outdoors and soak up the fresh air and sunshine.

Sleep Optimization

Getting enough quality sleep is essential for overall health and well-being, including weight management and metabolism. Below are some of the sleep optimization strategies:

1. Establish a Bedtime Routine
 - Formulate a relaxing bedtime routine to signal to your body that it's time to prepare for sleep.
 - Activities such as reading, taking a warm bath, or practicing relaxation techniques can help promote better sleep.

2. Create a Sleep-Friendly Environment
 - Make your bedroom sleep conducive by keeping it cool, dark, and quiet.
- Purchase a cozy mattress and pillows, and think about using blackout curtains or a white noise machine if necessary.

3. Limit Screen Time Before Bed
 - The blue light from screens can disrupt the production of melatonin, the hormone responsible for regulating sleep.

- Try to limit screen time to at least an hour before bed, and consider using blue light filters on your devices.

4. Avoid Caffeine and Alcohol Before Bed
- Caffeine and alcohol can disrupt sleep patterns and interfere with the quality of your sleep.
- Endeavor to avoid caffeine and alcohol especially in the hours leading up to bedtime.

5. Stick to a Consistent Sleep Schedule
-Maintain a consistent sleep routine by going to bed and waking up at the same time each day, including weekends.
- Consistency is crucial for regulating your body's internal clock and improving sleep quality.

Strategies for Long-Term Success

Committing to a healthy weight and lifestyle is a long-term endeavor. Below are some long term success strategies:

1. Set Realistic Goals
- Set achievable, realistic goals that you can work towards over time.

- Set big goals, and break them down into smaller, more manageable steps.

2. Focus on Consistency, Not Perfection
- Consistency is vital when you want to make lasting changes.
- Focus on making small, sustainable changes to your diet and exercise habits rather than trying to be perfect all the time.

3. Find What Works for You
- Experiment with different diet and exercise strategies to find what works best for your body and lifestyle.
- Everyone is unique, what works for another person may not work for you.

4. Practice Self-Compassion
- Be kind to yourself and practice self-compassion, especially when things don't go as planned.
- Remember that setbacks are a normal part of the journey, and it's okay to ask for help when you need it.

5. Stay Flexible and Adapt
- Life is unpredictable, and there will inevitably be obstacles and challenges along the way.

- Stay flexible and be willing to adapt your plan as needed to stay on track towards your goals.

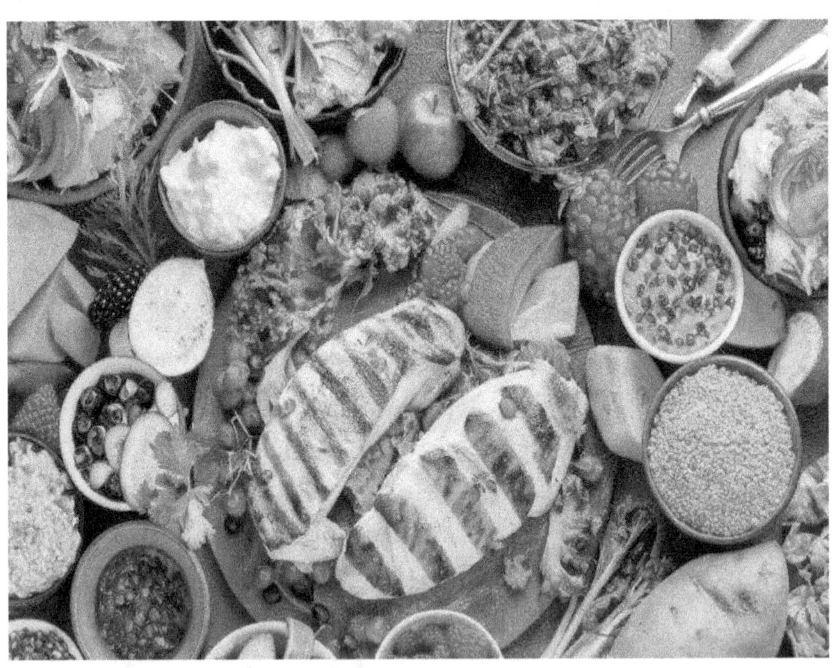

CONCLUSION

As an endomorph, achieving and maintaining a healthy weight and lifestyle may present unique challenges, but with the right approach, it's entirely possible.

Endomorphs typically have a slower metabolism, which may make it easier for them to gain weight and more challenging to lose it.

Genetics, hormones, muscle mass, diet, exercise habits, and age all play a role in metabolism and body composition.

Focus on a balanced diet that includes lean proteins, complex carbohydrates, healthy fats, fruits, and vegetables. Portion control is also essential, and it's crucial to pay attention to hunger and fullness cues.

Incorporate both cardiovascular exercise and strength training into your routine to support metabolism, burn calories, and build muscle. Mix up your workouts to keep your body challenged and avoid plateaus.

Manage stress through techniques such as exercise, deep breathing, mindfulness, and spending time in nature. Optimize your sleep by establishing a bedtime routine, creating a sleep-friendly environment, and sticking to a consistent sleep schedule.

Next Steps for Your Endomorph Journey

Now that you have a better understanding of your body type and the strategies that can help you achieve your health and fitness goals, set achievable, realistic goals for yourself, whether it's losing a certain amount of weight, improving your fitness level, or adopting healthier habits.

Develop a comprehensive plan that includes balanced nutrition, regular exercise, stress management techniques, and strategies for optimizing sleep. Consistency is very important when it comes to making lasting changes.

Keep track of your progress by monitoring your weight, measurements, fitness level, and how you feel both physically and mentally.

Be willing to adjust your plan as needed based on your progress, changing goals, and any obstacles or challenges that may arise.

Don't be afraid to reach out for support from friends, family members, or professionals if you need it. A support partner can help keep you motivated and accountable.

Remember, your journey as an endomorph is unique to you, and what works for someone else may not work for you. Stay patient, remain focused on your goals, and celebrate your progress as you go. With dedication and persistence, you can reach your health and fitness objectives and lead a happier, healthier life.